.

FIRST
RESPONDERS
in Love

NAVIGATING RELATIONSHIPS
IN HIGH-STRESS CAREERS

VANESSA KENNEDY

KP PUBLISHING COMPANY

ISBN: 978-1-960001-31-3 (Paperback)
ISBN: 978-1-960001-32-0 (Ebook)
Library of Congress Control Number: Pending

Editor: Stacie Fuji
Cover Design: Juan Roberts, Creative Lunacy
Literary Director: Sandra Slayton James

Published by:

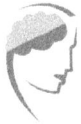

KP Publishing Company
Publisher of Fiction, Nonfiction & Children's Books
www.kp-pub.com

Printed in the United States of America

Introduction

Being a first responder is a demanding and rewarding career, but it can also affect personal relationships. The unique challenges of the job, including long hours, trauma exposure, and unpredictable schedules, can stress even the strongest of partnerships.

First responders, including firefighters, police officers, paramedics, and others, play a crucial role in keeping our communities safe. They put their lives on the line daily to respond to emergencies and save lives. However, being a first responder is physically demanding and emotionally taxing.

Navigating a relationship can be complex and challenging for first responders and their partners, but with the proper support and understanding, first-responder relationships can be strong, resilient, and fulfilling. This book aims to provide first responders and their partners with the tools and strategies they need to navigate the unique challenges of this high-stress career.

We will explore the challenges that first responders face in their relationships, including trauma exposure, the effects of shift work on personal lives, and the importance of effective communication. We will also discuss the steps that first responders and their partners can take to build a solid foundation for their relationship, including setting boundaries, prioritizing self-care, and fostering open and honest communication.

We will address the importance of seeking support, including therapy, support groups, and peer support programs. First responders and their partners can build a solid, loving relationship that can withstand job demands by understanding and developing the skills to overcome the unique challenges that come with this career.

Whether you are just starting a relationship with a first responder or have been together for years, this book offers practical and compassionate advice for building a solid and fulfilling partnership.

Contents

Introduction   *v*

Quiz   *ix*

Chapter 1:   Understanding the Challenges of
First Responder Relationships   1

Chapter 2:   Building a Strong Foundation
for Your Relationship   19

Chapter 3:   Code Red in the Bedroom—
Having a Healthy Sex Life   47

Chapter 4:   Balancing Work and Personal Life   77

Chapter 5:   Seeking Support When You Need It   101

Chapter 6:   Prioritizing Self-Care   117

Chapter 7:   Seeking Support   127

Chapter 8:   Maintaining Open Communication   133

Chapter 9:   Coping with Trauma Exposure   139

Chapter 10:   Coping Strategies for First Responders   159

              Conclusion   *161*

              Final Thoughts   *163*

              A Note from the Author   *169*

              About the Author   *171*

              References   *175*

Welcome to the First Responder Relationship Strength Quiz!

As a first responder, you face unique challenges balancing your demanding career and personal life. By taking this quiz, you will gain insight into the areas of your relationship that might need more attention and focus. Through self-reflection and open communication with your significant other, you can work together to build a stronger, more resilient partnership that withstands the pressures of your career. Remember, this quiz is a tool for self-assessment and growth—use the results to initiate conversations, identify areas for improvement, and foster a healthier, more supportive relationship with your loved one.

FIRST RESPONDER RELATIONSHIP STRENGTH QUIZ

Instructions: First responders face unique challenges when maintaining a healthy relationship with their significant other. Answer the following questions as honestly as possible to assess the strength of your relationship. For each question, choose the option that best describes your current situation.

How often do you communicate openly and honestly with your significant other about your feelings, thoughts, and concerns?

A) Almost always.

B) Most of the time.

C) Sometimes.

D) Rarely.

How well do you and your significant other manage and resolve conflicts?

A) We resolve conflicts effectively and calmly.

B) We mostly resolve conflicts but sometimes struggle.

C) We have difficulty resolving conflicts and often argue.

D) Conflicts often go unresolved and cause tension.

How supportive is your significant other in your career as a first responder?

A) Extremely supportive and understanding.

B) Supportive, but with occasional concerns.

C) Somewhat supportive but often expresses worries.

D) Not supportive and regularly critical.

Despite your demanding work schedule, how often do you and your significant other make time for each other?

A) We prioritize spending quality time together regularly.

B) We try to be available for each other, but it can be challenging.

C) We occasionally spend quality time together, but it is rare.

D) We only spend a little quality time together due to our schedules.

How well do you balance your relationship, work, and personal needs?

A) We balance our relationships, work, and personal needs effectively.

B) We mostly balance our needs, but it is a challenge.

C) We need help to balance our relationships, work, and personal needs.

D) We cannot balance our relationship, work, and personal needs.

How often do you express appreciation and gratitude towards each other?

A) Almost always.

B) Most of the time.

C) Sometimes.

D) Rarely.

How satisfied are you with the level of trust, intimacy, and emotional connection in your relationship?

A) Extremely satisfied.

B) Mostly satisfied.

C) Somewhat satisfied.

D) Not satisfied at all.

After completing the quiz, tally your scores for each response: A=4, B=3, C=2, D=1. Add up your total score to determine the strength of your relationship with your significant other:

28–24: Your connection is solid! Keep up the great work maintaining open communication, support, and trust with your significant other.

23–17: Your relationship is strong, but there is room for improvement. Work on improving communication, addressing concerns, and spending quality time together.

16–10: Your relationship may be facing some challenges. Prioritize open communication and mutual support to help strengthen your bond.

9–7: Your relationship is in a difficult stage. It is crucial to seek professional help, such as couples counseling, to address the issues and work on rebuilding trust and connection.

ASSESSMENT QUIZ

First Responder Therapy Assessment Quiz

Instructions: As a first responder, you face numerous challenges and stressors that can affect your mental health. This quiz will help you evaluate whether you may benefit from therapy. Answer each question honestly, choosing the option that best reflects your feelings and experiences. Please remember that this quiz is not a diagnostic tool but a starting point for self-reflection.

How often do you experience feelings of sadness, anxiety, or hopelessness?

A) Rarely.

B) Occasionally.

C) Frequently.

D) Almost all the time.

How well do you manage your stress levels related to your work as a first responder?

A) I manage stress effectively and maintain a healthy balance.

B) I manage stress reasonably well but sometimes struggle.

C) I have difficulty managing my stress and often feel overwhelmed.

D) I am constantly overwhelmed by stress and unable to cope.

How often do you have difficulty sleeping due to work-related thoughts or experiences?

A) Rarely.

B) Occasionally.

C) Frequently.

D) Almost all the time.

Have you experienced any traumatic events during your work as a first responder that continue to impact you?
- A) No, I haven't experienced any traumatic events.
- B) I've experienced traumatic events, but they do not affect me much.
- C) I've experienced traumatic events and sometimes struggle with the aftermath.
- D) I've experienced traumatic events that continue negatively impacting my life.

How often do you experience irritability, anger, or mood swings that affect your relationships or daily life?
- A) Rarely.
- B) Occasionally.
- C) Frequently.
- D) Almost all the time.

How often do you use unhealthy coping mechanisms (e.g., excessive drinking, substance abuse, overeating) to deal with work-related stress?
- A) Rarely.
- B) Occasionally.
- C) Frequently.
- D) Almost all the time.

Have friends, family members, or colleagues expressed concern about your mental health or well-being?
- A) No, no one has expressed concern.
- B) Rarely, but I believe it is under control.
- C) Occasionally, it has made me think about my mental health.
- D) Yes, frequently, and I am concerned as well.

After completing the quiz, tally your scores for each response: A=1, B=2, C=3, D=4. Add up your total score to determine whether seeking therapy might be beneficial for you:

7–12: Your mental health seems to be in a stable state. Continue to practice self-care and maintain a healthy work-life balance. However, be aware of any changes in your mental health and seek help if needed.

13–20: You may be experiencing some challenges with your mental health. It could be helpful to seek therapy or talk to a trusted friend or colleague about your feelings.

21–28: Your work as a first responder may significantly impact your mental health. Seeking therapy is highly recommended to help you cope with stress, trauma, and other challenges.

CHAPTER 1

Understanding the Challenges of First Responder Relationships

This chapter will explore the challenges first responders face in their relationships due to the demands of their jobs. This chapter will dive into these challenges in more detail and explore how they can impact a relationship. We will cover topics such as trauma exposure, the effects of shift work on personal lives, the importance of effective communication, stress management, lack of support, secondary trauma, lack of predictability, public perception, physical demands, and emotional distance.

TRAUMA EXPOSURE

One of the biggest challenges of being a first responder is the continuous or daily exposure to traumatic events. Trauma exposure is the experience of witnessing or being directly involved in a traumatic event, such as a natural disaster, accident, or act of violence.

Such exposure can affect a person's mental and emotional well-being and negatively affect their relationships. First responders may struggle with symptoms such as anxiety, depression, and PTSD, making it difficult to connect with their partners.

Trauma exposure can lead to multiple symptoms, including irritability, difficulty concentrating, forgetfulness, and confusion. Repeated exposure to traumatic events can lead to compassion fatigue and vicarious traumatization, further impacting an individual's mental and emotional well-being.

First responders must seek support and engage in self-care practices to cope with the impact of trauma exposure. This may involve seeking professional help, engaging in mindfulness practices, focusing on physical health, and building a solid support system. By seeking support and prioritizing self-care, first responders can improve their overall well-being and better cope with the effects of trauma exposure.

It is important to note that everyone reacts differently to trauma exposure, and the impact of trauma exposure can vary from person to person. Some individuals experience symptoms immediately after a traumatic event, while others experience symptoms years later. Some individuals may experience severe and long-lasting symptoms, while others may experience mild and short-lived symptoms.

Trauma exposure can also significantly impact first responders' relationships and family life. It is not uncommon for first responders to experience difficulties in their relationships, such as communication problems, conflict, and decreased intimacy. It is essential for first responders and their partners to understand the impact of trauma exposure and to seek support when needed.

To cope with the effects of trauma exposure, first responders may seek support from peer support programs, as connecting with others who understand the specific challenges of their job can be incredibly beneficial.

It is also crucial for first responders to educate themselves about the impact of trauma exposure and to understand the symptoms that may occur. This can help first responders to recognize when they may be experiencing the effects of trauma exposure and to seek support when needed. It is also crucial for first responders to understand that seeking help is a sign of strength, not weakness. Seeking help from a licensed therapist or counselor can provide first responders with the support and resources they need to cope. Seeking professional help, first responders can also engage in self-care practices, such as exercise, mindfulness, and relaxation techniques. Self-care practices can help first responders manage stress and improve their overall well-being.

First responders must contact their loved ones and build a dynamic support system. This may involve connecting with family, friends, and peers who understand the challenges of the job. By creating a solid support system, first responders can have a network of individuals to turn to when they need support and encouragement.

First responders are exposed to traumatic events as part of their job, and it is essential for them to understand the impact of trauma exposure and to seek support when needed. By prioritizing self-care, seeking professional help, and building a solid support system, first responders can improve their overall well-being and better cope with the effects of trauma exposure.

SHIFT WORK

First responders often work long and irregular hours, challenging maintaining a healthy work-life balance. This can lead to feelings of exhaustion and burnout, which can impact a relationship. Shift work can make it difficult for first responders and their partners to spend quality time together. Shift work refers to a work schedule that involves working outside the traditional 9 a.m.-5 p.m. workday. This can include working overnight shifts, rotating shifts, or working weekends. Shift work is standard in many industries, including healthcare, manufacturing, and law enforcement. For first responders, shift work is a regular part of their job, as they are often required to work irregular hours to respond to emergencies and keep our communities safe. However, shift work can significantly impact an individual's physical and mental health, as well as their relationships and family life.

The effects of shift work can include disrupted sleep patterns, fatigue, and difficulty sleeping, leading to decreased productivity, decreased mental and physical performance, and an increased risk of accidents and injuries. Shift work can also increase stress, reduce morale, and lower job satisfaction.

To cope with the effects of shift work, it is crucial for first responders to prioritize their physical and mental health and to engage in self-care practices. This may involve establishing a consistent sleep schedule, engaging in physical activity, and seeking professional help. It is also crucial for first responders to seek support from their loved ones and to build a dynamic support system. This may involve connecting with family, and working as a first responder may significantly impact your mental health.

Effective communication is critical to any successful relationship, especially for first responders. The stress of the job can make it difficult for first responders to communicate effectively with their partners, leading to misunderstandings and conflict. Communication is a fundamental aspect of any relationship and is especially important for first responders and their partners. The demands of the first responder job, including long hours, irregular schedules, and exposure to traumatic events, can place significant stress on a relationship and make open and effective communication even more critical.

Effective communication involves actively listening to each other, expressing oneself clearly and respectfully, and being open to feedback and different perspectives. Open communication can help first responders and their partners better understand each other's needs and concerns, resolve conflicts, and build a stronger, more fulfilling relationship.

Establishing ground rules for communication is essential in building a solid and effective communication style. This may involve setting aside regular time for open and honest discussions, avoiding blaming or criticism, and actively listening to each other's perspectives.

It is also crucial for first responders and their partners to be aware of the impact of trauma exposure on communication and to seek professional help when needed. Trauma exposure can lead to changes in behavior and emotions and can impact the ability to communicate effectively with others. Seeking professional help can provide first responders and their partners with the support and resources they need to improve their communication skills and build stronger, more fulfilling relationships.

Communication is critical to any relationship and essential for first responders and their partners. By establishing ground rules for communication, prioritizing open and effective communication, and seeking professional help when needed, first responders and their partners can build a solid and fulfilling relationship, even in the face of the unique challenges of the first responder job.

STRESS

First responders are often exposed to high levels of stress on the job, which can take a toll on their personal lives. This stress can impact their relationships, leading to irritability, anger, and frustration. Stress is a normal part of life, but it can become overwhelming when chronic. Chronic stress can lead to various physical and mental health problems, including anxiety, depression, irritability, fatigue, and difficulty sleeping. Stress is a significant issue for first responders, as the job demands can lead to chronic stress. Exposure to traumatic events, long hours, and irregular schedules can increase first responders' stress levels.

Below, Officer Davis shares his story of how he dealt with Stress.

Officer Jeremy Davis had always been a man of steel, both in physique and spirit. For over a decade, he had served his community with pride as a police officer. He was the first to arrive at the scene of accidents, violent crimes, and disturbances. He was known for his ability to remain calm under pressure, and his composure was a beacon of hope for those in need. Beneath his iron-clad exterior, the constant exposure to chaos started wearing him down.

Jeremy's wife, Sophie, noticed the change first. The once vibrant, jovial man who would race their kids around the backyard now appeared tired and distant. He was becoming irritable and quick-tempered, often snapping over trivial issues. The light that used to shine in his eyes seemed to dim each day. Their conversations about work were no longer about the people he had helped but about the traumatic events he had witnessed. Sophie knew this change was more than just fatigue; it reflected his chronic stress.

One day, Jeremy received a distress call about a major accident. He arrived at the scene to find a horrifying tableau of twisted metal and scattered debris. Amidst the chaos, he noticed a little girl, no older than his daughter, crying uncontrollably next to a wrecked car. It was a scene that broke even the toughest of hearts. That night, Jeremy couldn't sleep. The image of the terrified little girl was etched in his mind, triggering an avalanche of suppressed emotions. He woke up in a cold sweat, heart pounding, and it dawned on him that he needed help.

Acknowledging that he was struggling was not easy for a man known to be a pillar of strength. He felt it might be perceived as a sign of weakness, but he knew he owed it to himself and his family. He decided to reach out to the department's psychologist. Dr. Allen, the psychologist, was an empathetic listener. He reassured Jeremy that his feelings were completely normal, given his constant exposure to high-stress situations. He introduced Jeremy to "resilience training," which involved mindfulness exercises, cognitive behavioral techniques, and physical activities to reduce stress. The goal was not to eliminate stress but to learn how to handle it effectively.

With the support of Dr. Allen, Sophie, and his fellow officers, Jeremy began his journey toward managing his chronic stress. He began to meditate, practicing mindfulness to stay present and disconnect from the traumas of his job. He was taught to recognize his stress signals and respond to them proactively. Slowly but surely, Jeremy found himself regaining his lost energy. The irritability lessened; he slept better and felt more at ease.

The transformation was not overnight, but the change was evident. His colleagues noticed a calmer, more focused Jeremy. Sophie saw glimpses of the man she fell in love with returning. Their children noticed their dad's laughter echoing in their home once again. The journey was not easy, but Officer Davis stood as a testament that even the strongest among us could falter under chronic stress, and seeking help was not a weakness but a strength. It reminded his fellow first responders that it was okay to acknowledge their focus and manage it effectively to keep serving their communities with the same vigor and resilience.

When first responders don't have the support they need, they often experience feelings of isolation and loneliness. They can feel as if no one understands what they're going through. These feelings can be powerful if they're dealing with the after-effects of a traumatic event, such as a major accident or violent crime, and they don't have anyone to talk to about their experiences. This lack of support can lead to a significant increase in stress, anxiety, and depression. First responders may resort to unhealthy coping mechanisms without a safe outlet for their feelings, such as excessive drinking, substance use, or reckless behavior. These coping mechanisms can further exacerbate their feelings of stress and isolation.

The absence of support also creates a significant barrier to seeking help. First responders often worry about the stigma of seeking mental health assistance, particularly in professions that strongly emphasize being tough and resilient. They may fear admitting their struggles will make them appear weak or unfit for their job. They also often have a heightened sense of responsibility and guilt. If they're not at their best, they worry that they won't be able to effectively perform their duties, which could put people's lives at risk. This can create a vicious cycle, where the fear of being unable to do their job amplifies their stress, making it more difficult for them to do their job.

The lack of support also impacts their personal lives. Their family and friends may not fully understand their stress, leading to disconnect and tension in their relationships. Without help, they can feel as if they're carrying the weight of their job alone, which can cause strain on their relationships and lead to further feelings of isolation. The lack of support can make the already challenging job of a first responder even more difficult. It can lead to hopelessness and exhaustion and significantly impact their mental and emotional well-being.

However, they can break this cycle by seeking support from peer support programs, mental health professionals, and loved ones and improving their overall well-being.

LET'S TALK ABOUT PRIMARY AND SECONDARY TRAUMA.

Primary and secondary trauma, both significant in the mental health field, particularly for first responders, have distinct differences.

Primary trauma, often simply called trauma, is a term used to describe the psychological distress experienced after encountering a life-threatening or severely distressing event directly. Examples of events that can lead to primary trauma include physical or sexual assault, being in a severe accident, a natural disaster, victimless violence, or death. This trauma can lead to post-traumatic stress disorder (PTSD) and other mental health issues.

Secondary trauma, on the other hand, is a phenomenon where an individual experiences trauma symptoms not from exposure to a traumatic event but from hearing about or helping others navigate their traumatic experiences. Also known as vicarious trauma or compassion fatigue, it's common among individuals in helping professionals such as therapists, social workers, and first responders. They are often exposed to detailed accounts of traumatic events and their aftermath, which can impact their emotional well-being over time.

Secondary trauma can lead to symptoms like primary trauma, including hyperarousal, intrusive thoughts, and avoidance behaviors. Additionally, people suffering from secondary trauma can experience changes in their worldview, such as a heightened sense of danger or a decreased sense of safety, a sense of helplessness, or a reduced capacity to trust others.

While primary and secondary trauma sources differ, the impact on an individual's mental health can be equally profound. It's essential for individuals at risk of both primary and secondary trauma to be aware of the signs and symptoms and to seek professional help if needed.

LACK OF PREDICTABILITY

The unpredictable nature of a first responder's job can make it challenging to plan and prioritize personal and family time. This can lead to frustration and resentment, which can strain a relationship. Lack of predictability can be a significant source of stress for first responders, as the unpredictable nature of their jobs can make it challenging to plan their schedules and maintain a stable work-life balance. First responders are everyday heroes. They continually face unique challenges in their line of work. Let me illustrate with a personal story that helps put a human face on these incredible individuals.

John, a paramedic in a bustling city, works long and unpredictable hours. His days are filled with high-pressure, high-stakes situations requiring a calm demeanor, quick thinking, and deep empathy. One moment, he might comfort a scared child with a broken arm. The next, he could perform life-saving CPR on an elder with a heart attack. The unpredictability is exhausting, yet it's what John signed up for. It's his calling. One of John's most significant challenges in his job is maintaining a robust and healthy relationship with his wife, Sarah, and their two children. The long, unpredictable hours often mean missed family dinners, school recitals, and date nights.

In response, John and Sarah have devised some strategies to handle his schedule's irregularity and keep their relationship healthy and strong. They make communication a priority. Even when John is working, they exchange text messages throughout the day and make it a point to connect on video calls whenever there's a break in John's shift. Although initially uncomfortable with John's job's erratic nature, Sarah has become a pillar of support. She took the time to understand the stress and unpredictability of John's work. They regularly have open conversations about how they're feeling, and if a tough call is particularly affecting John, Sarah is there to listen and provide emotional support.

They also prioritized time together as a family. When John is off duty, they engage in activities that help them reconnect as a family, such as going on hikes, having family game nights, or simply sitting down for a family meal. These times provide the vital respite John needs from his high-stakes job and help him recharge.

Having family support, John actively participates in a peer support program offered by his department. This is a safe space where he can share his experiences and challenges with others who understand what it's like to be in his shoes. It's an essential part of his mental health toolkit.

John also prioritizes self-care. He's an early riser, dedicating an hour each morning to physical activity, such as running or yoga, before his shift begins. This keeps him physically fit and helps him clear his mind and prepare for the day. He has regular check-ins with a mental health professional, understands the importance of a sound sleep routine, and balances his diet, knowing that his job requires him to be in optimal health at all times. Being a first responder means living with unpredictability. But with a supportive spouse, open communication, peer support, and self-care practices, John and many other first responders are not just surviving in their careers—they're thriving. They're real-life superheroes, tackling each day and its unique challenges with strength, resilience, and dedication.

PUBLIC PERCEPTION

First responders often face public scrutiny and criticism, affecting their self-esteem and confidence. This can impact their relationships, leading to feelings of insecurity and doubt. Public perception of first responders can significantly impact their well-being, as negative stereotypes and misconceptions about their work can lead to frustration and disillusionment.

For example, some people may believe that first responders are immune to the effects of exposure to traumatic events or that they are not affected by the challenges of their job. This can lead to feelings of isolation and a lack of understanding from the public, which can harm first responders' mental and emotional well-being.

It is essential for first responders to educate the public about the realities of their job and to dispel common misconceptions. By sharing their experiences and educating the public about their challenges, first responders can help build a more accurate and understanding perception of their work.

Public perception of first responders can have a significant impact on their well-being. First, responders need to seek support and educate the public about the realities of their job. By doing so, first responders can improve their overall well-being and help to build a more accurate and understanding perception of their work.

PHYSICAL DEMANDS

First responders often engage in physically demanding activities on the job, which can lead to injury and exhaustion. This can impact their ability to participate in activities with their partners and strain relationships. The physical demands of being a first responder can be significant, as the job often requires physically demanding tasks and can lead to injury and burnout.

For example, first responders may be required to lift heavy equipment, perform CPR, and respond to emergencies in complex and potentially hazardous conditions. Over time, these physical demands can take a toll on a first responder's body, leading to injury and burnout. To understand the physical demands of their job, first responders need to prioritize their physical health and engage in self-care practices. This may involve engaging in regular physical activity, eating a healthy diet, and seeking medical attention when needed.

Let's continue to explore the importance of robust support systems, open communication, and peer support programs for first responders: Imagine Rachel, a firefighter working in a small town. Her job is physically demanding, with intense shifts involving fighting fires, rescuing people from dangerous situations, and providing emergency medical help. It's a career requiring peak physical fitness, mental toughness, and a deep dedication to her community. Rachel understands the importance of a solid support system and is fortunate to have her family and close friends standing by her. However, she knows that not all support must come from personal relationships. Hence, she turns to her second family—her team at the firehouse. They've formed a bond that only those who've faced the heat of a raging fire together can truly understand.

This camaraderie extends beyond the firehouse. They gather for regular cookouts where they can leave work behind and share laughter and stories. These times offer them a chance to decompress, and the understanding and mutual support they find in each other is invaluable. They don't have to explain the stress or physical exhaustion—each of them knows it all too well. Rachel also maintains open and honest communication with her partner, Alex. She makes it a point to express her feelings, particularly after a tough day. Alex may not understand the intricacies of her work, but he's there to lend a listening ear and a comforting presence. He's learned when to offer advice and when to hold her hand. Rachel commits to a rigorous workout routine to stay physically fit, even on her off days. She recognizes the importance of her physical well-being, not just for her job but for her overall health. To unwind, she enjoys long hikes with Alex, cherishing the serenity nature provides from the intensity of her work.

Rachel also actively engages in a peer support program organized by her town's first responder organizations. This group connects bi-weekly, discussing their experiences, sharing coping mechanisms, and reminding each other that seeking professional help is okay.

In this group, Rachel met Laura, a police officer, who became a close friend. They uniquely understand each other's experiences, offering mutual support during challenging times. Rachel and Laura also made it a point to participate in a mindfulness and meditation class together, another effective strategy they found for managing stress. Rachel's story shows you the power of robust support systems, open communication, self-care, and peer support in managing the physical demands and mental pressures of being a first responder. Her practices and methods demonstrate the essential combination of personal strength, communal support, and professional resources needed to thrive in this demanding career.

The physical demands of being a first responder can be significant. Still, they can be managed by prioritizing self-care, seeking professional help, building a solid support system, and seeking support from peer support programs. By taking these steps, first responders can improve their overall well-being and better cope with the physical demands of their job.

EMOTIONAL DISTANCE

Due to the nature of their job, first responders may struggle to maintain emotional closeness with their partners. They may feel disconnected and isolated, which can impact their relationship.

Kevin, an EMT, and Lily, a police officer, met during a joint training session for first responders. Their connection was immediate and intense. Amid the chaos and urgency of their jobs, they found in each other a calm harbor. Yet, the very nature of their careers, filled with stressful encounters and unpredictable schedules, often became a hurdle in their relationship. They had to face long periods apart, dealing with their emotional burdens alone. They often returned home exhausted, only to find their partner asleep or out on a call. They both deeply felt the isolation and disconnect creeping into their relationship.

During one tough week, Kevin was part of a team responding to severe car accidents. At the same time, Lily was involved in a high-stakes operation tracking down a dangerous criminal. They barely saw each other. The stress of their work, compounded by their emotional isolation, reached a tipping point. After another grueling shift, Kevin came home one evening to find Lily waiting for him. She had been granted a few hours off and had decided to use this time to address the growing chasm between them. They sat down and had a heart-to-heart conversation, expressing their feelings of disconnect, their longing for emotional closeness, and the challenges of their demanding jobs.

It was an emotionally charged evening filled with vulnerability and tears, but it marked a turning point in their relationship. They agreed to prioritize their connection, vowing to be there for each other emotionally, even when physically apart. They started to share their experiences more openly, even the most painful ones, becoming each other's safe space. They sent each other messages throughout the day, no matter how busy they were, to remind each other that they were in their thoughts. They started leaving notes for each other to find after long shifts, words of love and encouragement that reminded them of their bond.

In their rare, shared downtime, they invested in quality time together—a quiet walk in the park, cooking a meal together, or simply holding each other while watching a movie. They also sought professional counseling to better equip them with tools to handle their unique situation.

There were still challenging periods of disconnect, but they were now prepared to handle them. They had opened a channel of honest communication, recognized their emotional needs, and worked on fulfilling them.

Kevin and Lily's story serves as a heartwarming reminder of the power of connection and communication in overcoming the challenges of demanding careers like theirs. As first responders, they face high-stress, high-risk situations daily, but they learn to rely on each other, drawing strength from their bond, making their love story a valid showcase of resilience in the face of adversity.

First responders and their partners must understand the challenges they may face in their relationship. By being aware of these challenges and developing strategies to overcome them, first responders and their partners can build a robust and fulfilling relationship that can withstand the job demands. Emotional distance can be a common challenge for first responders, as their job needs can make maintaining close relationships with loved ones difficult. The experiences and challenges that first responders face are unique, and these experiences can significantly impact their emotional and mental state.

First responders are constantly exposed to traumatic incidents and crises. They witness pain, suffering, and sometimes death regularly. These experiences can leave deep imprints on their psyche, often leading to a condition called Vicarious Trauma, also known as Compassion Fatigue. This condition can cause feelings of sadness, anger, and helplessness, and in more severe cases, it can lead to symptoms like Post-Traumatic Stress Disorder (PTSD).

When they finish their shifts, first responders often carry these intense experiences home with them. They may find their thoughts frequently drifting back to incidents they attended, replaying distressing scenes, analyzing what they did, and wondering if they could have done anything differently. The "hero" label attached to first responders often exacerbates this. Society's expectation of them always being strong can make them feel as if they shouldn't show any signs of vulnerability, even to their loved ones. The fear of appearing weak or burdening their loved ones with their experiences often inhibits them from seeking support.

This can lead to emotional isolation and disconnection from others who may not fully understand what they're going through. Even with another first responder, like Kevin and Lily, they may hesitate to share their experiences and feelings, fearing it might add to their partner's stress. On top of the emotional stress, first responders also must deal with physical fatigue from working long, irregular hours and often under challenging conditions. This constant physical stress can add to their emotional strain, creating a cycle that can be hard to break without professional help. Yet, many first responders are reluctant to seek professional help due to fear of stigma, concern about their fitness for duty being questioned, or a deeply ingrained habit of trying to manage independently. They may also underestimate the impact of their experiences on their mental health until it starts affecting their relationships and overall well-being.

Understanding these internal struggles is crucial for supporting first responders. They must recognize that seeking help is not a sign of weakness but a step towards resilience. Support from loved ones, peer support programs, and professional mental health services can all play vital roles in helping them manage the psychological and emotional demands of their challenging careers.

In the next chapter, we will discuss the steps that first responders and their partners can take to build a strong foundation for their relationship, including setting boundaries, prioritizing self-care, and fostering open and honest communication. This foundation will provide a strong base for navigating the challenges of first responder relationships and building a lasting and loving partnership.

CHAPTER 2

Building a Strong Foundation for Your Relationship

This chapter will discuss the steps that first responders and their partners can take to build a strong foundation for their relationship. We will cover topics such as setting boundaries, prioritizing self-care, and fostering open and honest communication.

A strong foundation is essential for any successful relationship, and this is especially true for first-responder relationships. This chapter will discuss the steps that first responders and their partners can take to build a strong foundation for their relationship.

Setting Boundaries: First responders and their partners must set clear boundaries to separate their personal and work lives. This includes setting limits on work-related conversations at home, establishing a designated time for work-related phone calls, and finding ways to disconnect from work when at home. Setting boundaries is essential to managing the stress and challenges of being a first responder.

There are a variety of ways that first responders can set boundaries, including:

Defining work hours: First responders can explain their work hours and commit to not working outside of those hours unless it is an emergency.

Establishing clear communication with family and friends: First responders can communicate their work schedule and availability to loved ones and ensure they understand the importance of their job and the need for them to be available in an emergency.

Disconnecting from work: First responders can disconnect from work by turning off their phone or email notifications when off duty and engaging in activities that help them relax and recharge.

Seeking support from loved ones: First responders can seek consent from loved ones, who can provide emotional support and help them maintain a healthy work-life balance.

Setting boundaries is essential to managing the stress and challenges of being a first responder. By defining work hours, establishing clear communication with family and friends, disconnecting from work, and seeking support from loved ones, first responders can maintain a healthy work-life balance and improve their overall well-being.

PRIORITIZING SELF-CARE

First responders and their partners must prioritize self-care to maintain physical, mental, and emotional well-being. This includes exercising regularly, eating a healthy diet, getting enough sleep, and taking time for leisure activities. Prioritizing self-care is essential to managing the stress and challenges of being a first responder. Self-care refers to individuals' intentional and ongoing practices to maintain and improve their physical, emotional, and mental well-being.

There are a variety of self-care practices that first responders can engage in, including:

Exercise: Regular physical activity can help first responders manage stress, improve their physical health, and boost their mood.

Sleep: Getting enough sleep is essential for physical and mental well-being. First responders can prioritize sleep by establishing a consistent sleep schedule and creating a sleep-incentive environment.

Healthy eating: Eating a well-balanced diet can help first responders maintain their physical and mental health and provide them with the energy and nutrients they need to perform their job.

Relaxation and stress management techniques: Engaging in relaxation and stress management techniques, such as deep breathing, meditation, and yoga, can help first responders manage stress and improve their overall well-being.

Time with loved ones: Spending time with loved ones can provide first responders emotional support and help them maintain a healthy work-life balance.

Prioritizing self-care is essential to managing the stress and challenges of being a first responder. By engaging in regular self-care practices, first responders can improve their physical and mental well-being and better manage the demands of their job.

FOSTERING OPEN AND HONEST COMMUNICATION

Communication is critical to any successful relationship, and first-responder relationships are no exception. First responders and their partners must establish open and honest communication to ensure they are on the same page and avoid misunderstandings and conflict. Fostering open and honest communication is critical to maintaining healthy relationships among first responders. Open and honest communication can build trust and understanding between partners and provide a platform for addressing any challenges in the relationship.

There are several ways that first responders can foster open and honest communication, including:

Regular check-ins: Regular check-ins with partners can help ensure that both are on the same page and provide an opportunity for open and honest communication. Active listening: Active listening involves giving full attention to what your partner is saying and taking the time to understand their perspective. This can help to build trust and understanding in the relationship.

Avoiding assumptions: Avoiding assumptions and checking in with your partner can help to reduce misunderstandings and promote open and honest communication. Being transparent: Being transparent about your thoughts, feelings, and intentions can help to build trust and understanding in the relationship.

If communication challenges arise, seeking help from a therapist or relationship counselor can provide a safe and supportive environment for addressing these challenges. Fostering open and honest communication is critical to maintaining healthy relationships among first responders. By regularly checking in with partners, actively listening, avoiding assumptions, being transparent, and seeking outside help, if necessary, first responders can build solid and healthy relationships with their partners. First responders and their partners must support each other personally and professionally. This includes understanding each other's job demands, being there for each other during difficult times, and finding ways to have fun and enjoy each other's company. Supporting each other is crucial to maintaining healthy relationships for first responders. Support can come in many forms, from emotional support to practical assistance, and can help partners navigate the unique challenges of being a first responder.

There are several ways that first responders and their partners can support each other, including:

Emotional support: Emotional support can help partners manage stress and improve their well-being. This can involve being a sounding board, offering encouragement, and simply being there for each other when needed.

Practical support: Providing valuable support to each other can involve helping with daily tasks, such as grocery shopping or running errands, and can help partners manage the demands of their daily lives.

Encouragement: Encouraging each other in their personal and professional goals can help partners feel valued and supported and can help to build a solid and healthy relationship.

Taking time for each other: Taking time for each other, such as going on a date or engaging in a shared hobby, can help partners maintain a strong and healthy relationship.

Understanding each other's experiences: Understanding each other's experiences, such as the unique challenges and stressors of being a first responder, can help partners build a deeper understanding and connection. Supporting each other is crucial to maintaining healthy relationships for first responders. By providing emotional and practical support encouragement, taking time for each other, and understanding each other's experiences, first responders and their partners can build solid and healthy relationships that can withstand the unique challenges of being a first responder.

Seeking Outside Support: First responders and their partners may benefit from seeking outside support, such as therapy, support groups, or peer support programs. This can help them navigate the job's challenges and maintain a strong and healthy relationship. Seeking outside support is essential to maintaining healthy relationships for first responders. External support can come in many forms, from therapy to support groups. It can provide partners with the tools and resources to navigate the unique challenges of being a first responder.

There are several ways that first responders and their partners can seek outside support, including:
Therapy: Therapy can provide partners with a safe and supportive environment to address relationship challenges and improve communication and relationship skills.

Support groups: Support groups can provide partners with a community of individuals who understand the unique challenges of being a first responder and can provide a platform for sharing experiences and offering support.

Couples counseling: Couples counseling can provide partners with a safe and supportive environment to address relationship challenges and improve communication and relationship skills.

Mentorship programs: Mentorship programs can provide partners with a mentor who has experience as a first responder and can offer guidance and support.

Online resources: Online resources, such as websites and forums, can provide partners with information and resources to help them navigate the unique challenges of being a first responder.

Seeking outside support is essential to maintaining healthy relationships for first responders. By seeking therapy, support groups, couples counseling, and mentorship programs and utilizing online resources, first responders and their partners can build solid and healthy relationships and better manage the unique challenges of being a first responder.

ESTABLISHING SHARED GOALS AND VALUES

First responders and their partners must have a shared understanding of their goals and values to build a strong foundation for their relationship. This includes discussing their future, their priorities in life, and their individual and collective goals. Establishing shared goals and values is essential to maintaining healthy relationships among first responders. Shared goals and values provide partners with a shared vision for the future and a sense of purpose and bring partners closer together.

Open communication is crucial in establishing shared goals and values, allowing partners to discuss their hopes and aspirations for the future openly. Joint decision-making can help partners develop shared goals and values by involving both partners in decision-making. Engaging in shared activities, such as volunteering or participating in community events, can help partners to establish shared goals and values. Joint planning can help partners to develop shared goals and values by working together to plan. Aligning priorities, such as financial goals or family planning, can help partners to establish shared goals and values.

Establishing shared goals and values is essential to maintaining healthy relationships among first responders. First responders and their partners can build solid and healthy relationships based on shared ideals and values by engaging in open communication, joint decision-making, shared activities, collaborative planning, and aligning priorities.

BUILDING TRUST

Trust is the cornerstone of any strong relationship, and first-responder relationships are no exception. First responders and their partners must work to build and maintain trust through open and honest communication, supporting each other, and being there for each other through thick and thin. Building trust is a critical aspect of maintaining healthy relationships with first responders. Trust is the foundation of any solid and healthy relationship and can provide partners with security and stability.

Honesty is the cornerstone of trust; partners must be open and honest to build trust. Consistency in behavior and actions can help partners to build trust by demonstrating reliability and dependability. Open communication is critical to building trust and providing partners a platform for addressing challenges or concerns. Fulfilling commitments and meeting expectations can help partners build trust. Forgiving partners for mistakes and working through challenges can help them build confidence and strengthen their relationship.

Building trust is a critical aspect of maintaining healthy relationships with first responders. First responders and their partners can build solid and healthy relationships based on trust and mutual respect by being honest, consistent, engaging in open communication, fulfilling commitments, and forgiving.

MAINTAINING INTIMACY

The job demands can make it difficult for first responders to maintain intimacy in their relationships. First responders and their partners must prioritize intimacy and find ways to connect, such as through physical touch, shared experiences, or intimate conversations. Maintaining intimacy is an essential aspect of maintaining healthy relationships for first responders. Familiarity can provide partners with a sense of closeness and emotional connection and can help to strengthen the bond between partners.

Physical affection, such as holding hands or cuddling, can help partners to maintain intimacy and provide a sense of closeness. Spending quality time together, such as going on a date or engaging in a shared hobby, can help partners maintain intimacy. Open and honest communication can help partners maintain intimacy by providing a platform for addressing challenges or concerns. Sharing experiences, such as taking a trip or participating in a shared hobby, can help partners maintain intimacy and build a deeper connection. Engaging in intimate acts, such as sexual intimacy, can help partners to sustain intimacy and provide a sense of closeness.

Let's get into it. . . . The romantic story of Jack, a paramedic, and Maya, a firefighter.

They met at the scene of an apartment fire. Jack provided medical support while Maya was on the team fighting the fire. Amidst the chaos, they exchanged glances that sparkled with mutual respect and admiration.

They got to know each other better in the following weeks, their connection growing stronger with every shared cup of coffee, laugh, and every exchange of their challenging experiences. One fantastic evening, after a long, grueling day, Jack surprised Maya by turning up at her station with a bag full of takeout from her favorite Thai place. They shared dinner on the rooftop of the fire station, their conversation easy and their laughter echoing in the stillness of the night. It was the first time they had managed to relax together truly. As the stars twinkled above, Jack took Maya's hand, his touch sending warmth coursing through her. His gaze held a promise of understanding, shared burdens, and joys. He leaned in, and their lips met in a soft kiss, a seal of their budding romance. That moment of shared intimacy they have marked the beginning of their romantic relationship.

Their demanding jobs meant stolen kisses between shifts, hasty lunch dates, and hurried goodbyes. Despite the rush, each moment of shared intimacy was a precious reminder of their connection. They often stayed in bed on their rare days off, sharing stories, dreams, and fears. Their physical intimacy was an affirmation of their emotional bond, a way to express their feelings when words fell short.

One winter night, after an emotionally draining shift involving a particularly tragic incident, Maya came home to find Jack waiting for her, his concern evident in his eyes. He pulled her into his arms, holding her as she let the pent-up tears flow. He whispered words of comfort, reassurances that they were in this together. He understood her pain because he, too, had felt it. That night, they found solace in each other's arms, their shared intimacy a balm to their aching hearts. Through moments of joy and periods of hardship, Jack and Maya's relationship remained steadfast, their intimacy deepening with each shared experience. Their professions often asked much of them, but it also gave them something precious—a bond forged in the heat of chaos, a love resilient in the face of adversity. Their shared intimate moments were more than expressions of their physical desire; they reaffirmed their commitment, a sanctuary where they felt seen, understood, and loved.

The story of Jack and Maya exemplifies how first responders, despite the challenges of their careers, can foster deep romantic relationships. The key lies in shared moments of intimacy, both emotional and physical, which serve as an oasis amidst their demanding lives.

Maintaining intimacy is an essential aspect of maintaining healthy relationships for first responders. By engaging in physical affection, spending quality time together, open communication, sharing experiences, and intimate acts, first responders and their partners can maintain a solid and healthy relationship based on intimacy and emotional connection.

ENCOURAGING PERSONAL GROWTH:

First responders and their partners must encourage each other's personal growth and development. This includes supporting each other's interests and hobbies, promoting education and career development, and fostering a growth-oriented mindset. Encouraging personal growth is essential to maintaining healthy relationships for first responders. Personal growth can provide partners with a sense of purpose and fulfillment and can help to improve their overall well-being.

There are several ways that first responders and their partners can encourage personal growth, including:

Supporting personal goals: Supporting each other's dreams, such as education or career aspirations, can help partners encourage personal growth.

Encouraging personal development: Personal development, such as taking classes or pursuing new hobbies, can help partners encourage personal growth.

Encouraging: Encouragement and support can help partners pursue their personal goals and develop their skills and abilities.

Encouraging independence: Encouraging and encouraging partners to pursue their interests can help partners promote personal growth.

Celebrating accomplishments: Celebrating each other's achievements can help partners feel valued and supported and can help to encourage personal growth.

Encouraging personal growth is essential to maintaining healthy relationships for first responders. By supporting personal goals, encouraging personal development, providing encouragement, encouraging independence, and celebrating accomplishments, first responders and their partners can maintain a strong and healthy relationship that encourages personal growth and fulfillment.

CELEBRATING SUCCESSES

First responders and their partners must celebrate each other's successes, big or small. This can include recognizing each other's achievements, expressing gratitude for each other's contributions, and finding ways to celebrate each other's milestones. Celebrating successes is an essential aspect of maintaining healthy relationships for first responders. Celebrating successes provides partners with a sense of accomplishment and satisfaction and helps strengthen the bond between partners.

Recognizing and acknowledging each other's achievements, such as promotions or completing a complex project, can help partners celebrate successes. Celebrating milestones, such as anniversaries or birthdays, can help partners to celebrate successes and reflect on their achievements. Sharing each other's happiness and celebrating each other's successes can help partners to build a deeper connection and strengthen their bond. Celebrating successes, such as achieving a common goal or overcoming challenges, can help partners build stronger relationships. Creating special memories, such as taking a trip or having a special dinner, can help partners celebrate successes and build a stronger bond.

Celebrating successes is a critical aspect of maintaining healthy relationships for first responders. By recognizing accomplishments, celebrating milestones, sharing in each other's joy, celebrating as a team, and creating special memories, first responders and their partners can maintain a strong and healthy relationship that celebrates successes and builds a deeper bond.

ENCOURAGING POSITIVE COMMUNICATION

First responders and their partners must work to establish positive and respectful communication patterns in their relationships. This includes avoiding negative language, practicing active listening, and finding ways to express appreciation and gratitude for each other. Encouraging positive communication is essential to maintaining healthy relationships among first responders. Positive communication can give partners a sense of understanding and support and help build a stronger and more resilient relationship.

Active listening, where partners pay close attention to each other and show empathy, can help to encourage positive communication. Avoiding blame and instead focusing on finding solutions to problems can help promote positive communication. Using "I" statements: Using "I" statements, such as "I feel" or "I need," can help partners express their thoughts and feelings in a positive and non-confrontational manner. Avoiding negative communication patterns, such as criticism or sarcasm, can help to encourage positive communication. Encouraging open and honest dialogue, where partners feel comfortable expressing their thoughts and feelings, can help to promote positive communication.

Encouraging positive communication is essential to maintaining healthy relationships among first responders. First responders and their partners can maintain a solid and healthy relationship based on positive communication and mutual understanding by actively listening, avoiding blame, using "I" statements, avoiding negative communication patterns, and encouraging open and honest dialogue.

First responders and their partners can benefit from building a solid support system, including family, friends, and other community members. This support system can provide additional resources and support during difficult times and help strengthen the relationship. Building a solid support system is essential to maintaining healthy relationships among first responders. A robust support system can provide partners with a sense of security and stability and help them navigate the challenges they may face. Ethan and Grace tell their story of how important a support system is.

It all started in the bustling city of Chicago, where there lived a couple whose love was as intense and enduring as the fires that the husband, Ethan, fought as a first responder. Ethan was a dedicated firefighter, well-respected by his colleagues, while his wife, Grace, was a popular elementary school teacher. Their life together was a unique blend of Ethan's unpredictable shifts and the regular rhythm of Grace's school calendar. They relied heavily on their network of friends and family to keep their home life running smoothly. When Ethan was called for an emergency in the middle of the night, Grace's sister would rush over to stay with their two young children.

The couple was aware of the toll Ethan's profession could take on their relationship, so they prioritized their connection above all else. They always shared their highs and lows, dreams and fears with each other.

Grace had a calming presence that Ethan often relied on, especially after a particularly challenging day at work.

A few years into Ethan's career, he experienced a particularly traumatic event—a fire in which he was nearly trapped. He managed to escape, but the incident left a deep imprint on his psyche. He became more withdrawn and started having nightmares, the traumatic event haunting him day and night. Recognizing these signs, Grace encouraged Ethan to seek professional help. Though initially resistant, he agreed for her sake and started attending therapy sessions with a counselor who specialized in trauma. Grace was his pillar of strength, offering unconditional support and love. The therapy and Grace's enduring support helped Ethan understand and navigate his trauma.

During this challenging time, Grace also sought support outside their immediate family. She found a local support group for partners of first responders, where she could share her experiences and learn from others going through similar circumstances. This network provided much-needed support and understanding, giving Grace the strength to support Ethan.

As Ethan navigated his journey towards healing, Grace started incorporating mindfulness practices into their daily routine. She learned that resilience-building activities could help manage stress and improve overall well-being. They started meditating together, going for early morning runs, and practicing yoga, transforming their ordeal into an opportunity to strengthen their bond.

Over time, Ethan started showing signs of improvement. His nightmares decreased, and he became more open, sharing his fears and insecurities with Grace. Their relationship, tested by fire, emerged stronger. They became each other's rock, understanding and supporting each other in ways they hadn't before.

Their story became a true love story and showed the power of love, resilience, and the importance of a robust support system. Ethan, the brave firefighter, and Grace, the dedicated teacher, demonstrated that even when life brings a storm, a strong relationship can weather it and emerge stronger. They reminded their community that behind every first responder is a supporting partner, playing an equally important role, away from the frontlines but close to the heart.

Building a solid support system is essential to maintaining healthy relationships among first responders. By making a network of friends and family, joining a support group, seeking professional help, relying on each other, and building resilience, first responders and their partners can maintain a solid and healthy relationship supported by a robust support system.

FINDING SHARED HOBBIES AND INTERESTS.

First responders and their partners must find shared hobbies and interests to connect and build a strong bond. This can include participating in sports or fitness activities, traveling, or volunteering together. Finding shared hobbies and interests is essential to maintaining healthy relationships for first responders. Shared hobbies and interests provide partners with a sense of connection and shared experiences and strengthen the bond between partners.

There are several ways that first responders and their partners can find shared hobbies and interests, including:

Exploring new interests: Exploring new attractions together, such as trying a new sport or hobby, can help partners find shared hobbies and interests.

Participating in: Activities like cooking or gardening can help partners find shared hobbies and interests.

Encouraging each other's interests: Encouraging each other's interests, even if they are not shared, can help partners find shared hobbies and interests and build a deeper understanding of each other.

Joining a club or organization: Joining a club or organization that aligns with a shared interest can help partners find shared hobbies and interests and build a stronger bond.

Planning shared experiences: Planning shared experiences like taking a trip or attending a concert can help partners find shared hobbies and interests and build a stronger bond.

Finding shared hobbies and interests is essential to maintaining healthy relationships for first responders. First responders and their partners can maintain a strong and healthy relationship based on shared hobbies and interests by exploring new attractions, participating in shared activities, encouraging each other's interests, joining a club or organization, and planning shared experiences.

PRACTICING GRATITUDE.

First responders and their partners must practice gratitude and find ways to express appreciation for each other. This can include writing love letters, expressing gratitude during conversations, or simply taking the time to recognize each other's contributions to the relationship. Practicing gratitude is an essential aspect of maintaining healthy relationships for first responders. Gratitude can provide partners with a positive outlook and a sense of appreciation for each other and their relationship and can help strengthen the bond between partners.

There are several ways that first responders and their partners can practice gratitude, including:

Expressing gratitude: Expressing gratitude for each other and their relationship can help partners practice appreciation and build a stronger bond.

Keeping a gratitude journal: Keeping a gratitude journal and writing down things they are grateful for can help partners practice gratitude and focus on the positive aspects of their relationship.

Celebrating small victories: Celebrating small achievements, such as completing a task or overcoming a challenge, can help partners practice gratitude and appreciate each other's efforts.

Focusing on the present moment: Focusing on the present moment and appreciating the small things can help partners practice gratitude and build a stronger bond.

Encouraging acts of kindness: Encouraging acts of kindness, such as doing something special for each other, can help partners practice gratitude and build a stronger bond.

Practicing gratitude is essential to maintaining healthy relationships with first responders. First responders and their partners can maintain a solid and healthy relationship based on gratitude and appreciation by expressing gratitude, keeping a gratitude journal, celebrating small victories, focusing on the present moment, and encouraging acts of kindness.

BUILDING RESILIENCE.

First responders and their partners must build resilience in their relationship to withstand the challenges that come with the job. This can include establishing a solid support system, practicing self-care, and seeking support when needed.

Building resilience is an essential aspect of maintaining healthy relationships for first responders. Strength can help partners better cope with the stress and challenges they may face and can provide a foundation for a strong and healthy relationship.

There are several ways that first responders and their partners can build resilience, including:
Engaging in mindfulness practices: Engaging in mindfulness practices, such as meditation or yoga, can help partners to build resilience and manage stress.

Engaging in mindfulness practices is essential to building resilience and maintaining healthy relationships for first responders. Mindfulness practices, such as meditation or yoga, can help partners focus on the present moment, manage stress, and build a solid and healthy relationship.

There are several mindfulness practices that first responders and their partners can engage in, including:
Meditation: Meditation is a mindfulness practice that focuses on the present moment and letting go of distractions. Regular meditation can help partners to manage stress and build resilience.

Yoga is a mindfulness practice involving physical postures, breathing techniques, and meditation. Regular yoga practice can help partners to manage stress and build resilience.

Deep breathing: Deep breathing is a mindfulness practice that involves taking slow, deep breaths and focusing on the sensation of breathing. Regular deep breathing can help partners to manage stress and build resilience.

Guided imagery: Guided imagery is a mindfulness practice that involves imagining festive scenes and experiences to manage stress and build resilience.

Body scan meditation: Body scan meditation is a mindfulness practice that involves lying down or sitting and focusing on each part of the body, releasing tension, and promoting relaxation.

Engaging in mindfulness practices is essential to building resilience and maintaining healthy relationships for first responders. By incorporating meditation, yoga, deep breathing, guided imagery, or body scan meditation into their daily routine, first responders and their partners can manage stress, build resilience, and maintain a strong and healthy relationship.

Exercising regularly, such as walking or running, can help partners build resilience and manage stress.

Exercising regularly is essential to building resilience and maintaining healthy relationships for first responders. Regular exercise can help partners manage stress, build strength, and provide a foundation for a strong and healthy relationship.

There are several ways that first responders and their partners can exercise regularly, including:

Going for a walk or run: Going for a walk or run is a simple and effective way to exercise regularly and manage stress.

Participating in team sports: Team sports, such as basketball or soccer, can allow partners to exercise regularly and build a sense of camaraderie.

Taking fitness classes: Fitness classes like dance or spinning can give partners a fun and engaging way to exercise regularly and manage stress.

Hiking or camping: Hiking or camping can allow partners to exercise regularly and connect with nature.

Doing at-home workouts: Doing at-home activities, such as yoga or strength training, can allow partners to exercise regularly and manage stress in the comfort of their homes.

Exercising regularly is essential to building resilience and maintaining healthy relationships for first responders. First responders and their partners can manage stress, build strength, and maintain a strong and healthy relationship by walking or running, participating in team sports, taking fitness classes, hiking or camping, or doing at-home workouts.

GETTING ADEQUATE SLEEP

Getting adequate sleep is essential to building resilience and maintaining healthy relationships for first responders. Sufficient sleep can help partners manage stress, build strength, and provide a foundation for a strong and healthy relationship.

There are several ways that first responders and their partners can ensure they get adequate sleep, including:
Establishing a sleep routine: Going to bed and waking up simultaneously daily can help partners get adequate sleep.

Creating a sleep-conducive environment: A sleep-conducive climate, such as keeping the bedroom cool and dark, can help partners get adequate sleep.

Avoiding screens before bedtime: Avoiding screens, such as televisions, phones, and computers, before rest can help partners get adequate sleep.

Engaging in relaxing activities before bedtime: Engaging in relaxing activities, such as reading a book or taking a warm bath, before rest can help partners get adequate sleep.

Practicing good sleep hygiene: Good sleep hygiene, such as avoiding caffeine and alcohol before bedtime, can help partners get adequate sleep.

Getting adequate sleep is essential to building resilience and maintaining healthy relationships for first responders. By establishing a sleep routine, creating a sleep-conducive environment, avoiding screens before bedtime, engaging in relaxing activities before bedtime, and practicing good sleep hygiene, first responders and their partners can manage stress, build resilience, and maintain a strong and healthy relationship.

Eating a healthy diet: Eating a nutritious diet, such as incorporating fruits and vegetables into their meals, can help partners to build resilience and manage stress. Eating a healthy diet is essential to building resilience and maintaining healthy relationships for first responders. A healthy diet can help partners manage stress, build strength, and provide a foundation for a strong and healthy relationship.

There are several ways that first responders and their partners can eat a healthy diet, including:

Incorporating fruits and vegetables into their meals: Incorporating fruits and vegetables into their meals can provide partners with essential vitamins, minerals, and fiber.

Limiting processed foods: Limiting processed foods like chips and candy can help partners avoid unhealthy sources of added sugars and saturated fats.

Choosing lean proteins: Lean proteins, such as chicken or fish, can help partners maintain a healthy weight and build muscle.

Incorporating healthy fats into their diet: Healthy fats, such as avocados and nuts, can help partners maintain a healthy weight and reduce the risk of heart disease.

Drinking plenty of water: Drinking plenty of water can help partners to stay hydrated and maintain a healthy weight.

Eating a healthy diet is essential to building resilience and maintaining healthy relationships for first responders. By incorporating fruits and vegetables into their meals, limiting processed foods, choosing lean proteins, incorporating healthy fats into their diet, and drinking plenty of water, first responders and their partners can manage stress, build resilience, and maintain a strong and healthy relationship.

Seeking professional help: Professional help, such as counseling or therapy, can provide partners with the tools and resources they need to build resilience and manage stress.

Seeking professional help is essential to building resilience and maintaining healthy relationships for first responders. Professional service can provide partners the support and resources they need to manage stress, build strength, and maintain a strong and healthy relationship. Leo's story tells us that change can happen for even the hardest of them all.

In the city of San Francisco lived a first responder named Leo. Leo was a seasoned police officer, well-known for his stern demeanor and no-nonsense attitude. He was revered by his peers and feared by the criminals he apprehended. Leo's life revolved around his work, his dedication sometimes coming at the expense of his personal life. Leo had always been a man rooted in logic and reality. He had a saying: "I believe in what I can see and touch." This was his motto, extending from his professional life to his personal beliefs. As such, he was deeply skeptical about anything he considered 'mystical' or 'otherworldly,' like therapy, which he called "wizardry."

However, an intense hostage situation that Leo managed to resolve but nearly cost him his life triggered a shift in his otherwise stable world. Nightmares filled his sleep, anxiety shadowed his every move, and the confidence he once possessed seemed to waver. His relationships started to suffer as he became more withdrawn, his skepticism of therapy as a barrier to seeking help.

His partner at the precinct, Dana, noticed Leo's struggle. She suggested he consider counseling or therapy. Leo scoffed at the idea, calling therapists "wizards who mess with your mind." Understanding his skepticism, Dana told him, "Sometimes, Leo, even the strongest warriors need a wizard."

Despite his initial resistance, the persistence of his symptoms and Dana's gentle nudging led Leo to reconsider his stance. He finally decided to try therapy, figuring he had nothing to lose.

The 'wizard' he met was a woman named Dr. Amelia, a therapist specializing in trauma. Over many sessions, Dr. Amelia helped Leo discover the root of his anxieties, teaching him coping strategies and offering insights that Leo reluctantly began to accept as logical and helpful.

Dr. Amelia used cognitive-behavioral therapy to help Leo confront his fears and manage his stress. He learned how to recognize and challenge his negative thought patterns and how to cope with his trauma-related anxieties. The process was not easy; Leo sometimes wanted to quit, but he persevered, driven by the subtle changes he started noticing in himself. Leo's perspective began to shift. He realized that therapy wasn't 'wizardry' but a tool, a lifeline that allowed him to regain control over his life. He started sleeping better, improved his mood, and slowly regained his lost confidence. His relationships, especially with his partner Dana, strengthened as he learned to express his feelings and fears.

His attitude towards his job also changed. Leo became more patient, empathetic, and effective in dealing with tense situations, applying the stress management strategies he learned from therapy. His peers noticed the change in him—the stern, rigid Leo had evolved into a more compassionate, understanding officer, respected for his courage and emotional intelligence.

Leo's journey to becoming a different and better man, both on the job and in his personal life, is a very proud moment, along with the power of seeking help. He realized that sometimes, the most substantial thing one can do is to admit they need help. Leo, once a skeptic of 'wizards,' became a firm believer in the power of therapy, understanding that resilience could be built and fears could be faced with the proper support and guidance. His story inspires many others in his line of work, showing them that seeking help isn't a sign of weakness but a step toward strength.

There are several types of professional help that first responders and their partners can seek, including:

Couples therapy: Couples therapy can allow partners to work through any relationship challenges they may be facing, build resilience, and maintain a strong and healthy relationship.

Individual therapy: Individual therapy can allow partners to work through any personal challenges they may be facing, build resilience, and maintain a strong and healthy relationship.

Group therapy: Allows partners to connect with others facing similar challenges, build resilience, and maintain a strong and healthy relationship.

Trauma-focused therapy: Can allow partners to work through any trauma they may have experienced, build resilience, and maintain a strong and healthy relationship.

PSYCHIATRIST OR PSYCHOLOGIST:

A psychiatrist or psychologist can provide partners with an opportunity to receive a comprehensive evaluation, build resilience, and maintain a strong and healthy relationship.

Seeking professional help is essential to building resilience and maintaining healthy relationships for first responders. First responders and their partners can manage stress, build strength, and maintain a strong and healthy relationship by seeking couples therapy, individual therapy, group therapy, trauma-focused therapy, or seeing a psychiatrist or psychologist.

Building resilience is an essential aspect of maintaining healthy relationships for first responders. By engaging in mindfulness practices, exercising regularly, getting adequate sleep, eating a healthy diet, and seeking professional help, first responders and their partners can maintain a solid and healthy relationship based on resilience and managing stress.

In the next chapter, we will delve into the specific challenge of trauma exposure and provide strategies for managing its effects on relationships. By understanding the impact of trauma and developing strategies to cope with it, first responders and their partners can build a strong, resilient, and fulfilling relationship.

CHAPTER 3

Code Red in the Bedroom— Having a Healthy Sex Life

Ready to take the heat from the streets to the sheets? If you're in love with a first responder, you already know the thrill of a life less ordinary. But did you know that spicing up your sexual connection can be the ultimate stress reliever for you both? Imagine lighting up your bedroom with the same urgency and passion they bring to saving lives.

The stakes are consistently elevated from the adrenaline-pumping highs to the soul-deep emotional lows. And when you're both giving it your all, body and soul, sparks don't just fly—they ignite in an all-consuming blaze of glory that can turn your love life into a pulse-pounding adventure. So why settle for routine when you can share in the same life-affirming rush that defines their calling? Dive into this chapter and discover how to reignite your sexual life in a way that truly honors the heroes that first responders are—in every aspect of their lives.

The job of a first responder is a call to action, a relentless commitment to saving lives and maintaining public safety. Amid this demanding lifestyle—filled with late-night shifts, high-stress scenarios, and a never-ending sense of responsibility—it can be easy to neglect one's well-being, especially concerning intimate relationships and sexual health.

Many first responders find that the pressures of their careers create unique challenges for maintaining a fulfilling sex life. This chapter addresses the often unspoken but vital issue of sex for first responders, focusing on navigating the intricacies of intimacy amidst a demanding job. Whether you're a firefighter, police officer, EMT, or military personnel, the information and advice shared here will help you understand the complexities and strategies for maintaining a healthy, satisfying sexual relationship while managing your profession's daily stressors and responsibilities.

We will be introduced to the impact of stress and adrenaline on your sex life, the importance of communication with your partner, and the role of emotional and physical health. Practical tips and expert advice will be offered to help you not just understand these challenges but to thrive despite them.

The subject of sex, often shrouded in taboo or awkwardness, deserves open discussion and attention, especially for those in roles that are emotionally and physically demanding. A solid sexual connection is not just beneficial but essential for the well-being and stability of long-term relationships, and it's time we start talking about it openly in the context of the high-stakes, high-stress world of first responders.

Let me share a quick story with you:

The Rekindled Flame:
A Case Study in Following Advice for a Healthy Sexual Relationship

Meet Emily and Jack, both first responders in a bustling city—Emily, a seasoned nurse, and Jack, a dedicated firefighter. The first few years of their marriage were filled with passion and intimacy. However, as their careers progressed, the irregular schedules, emotional toll, and exhaustion began to chip away at their once-flourishing sexual relationship. Date nights became a rarity, and moments of intimacy seemed more like obligatory chores rather than acts of love.

They both recognized something had to change, but how?

THE WAKE-UP CALL

Emily came across a book titled "First Responders in Love" and was particularly drawn to a chapter focused on sex and intimacy. Intrigued, she shared it with Jack, who was equally concerned about their dwindling passion. They both agreed to follow the advice and guidelines presented in the chapter, hoping for a change in their relationship dynamic.

Implementing the Advice: Addressing Stress: Emily and Jack began practicing mindfulness and relaxation exercises before bedtime to alleviate work-induced stress.

Open Communication: They set aside time each week to openly discuss their needs, desires, and any concerns in their sexual relationship, no holds barred.

Work-Life Balance: Despite their chaotic work schedules, they committed to setting aside time for intimacy, even if it meant planning weeks.

Health Checks: Both started routine medical examinations to rule out physical barriers to a satisfying sexual life.

Seeking Help: Jack, struggling with mild PTSD, took the advice from the chapter to seek therapy. This had a significant positive impact on his emotional availability and intimacy with Emily.

THE OUTCOME

Emily and Jack noticed a remarkable difference six months after implementing these changes. The quality of their intimate time improved exponentially. Emily felt more emotionally connected, enabling her to experience sexual pleasure more profoundly. Jack found his performance anxiety significantly reduced and his libido revitalized. Even their professional lives seemed to benefit from their newfound emotional well-being.

But the most significant change was invisible and intangible—yet palpable. It deepened their emotional connection, solidified by their shared commitment to maintaining a healthy sexual relationship. The passion they thought they had lost was now rekindled, not just reigniting their sex life but also fortifying their marriage.

Their journey isn't unique but is a testament to the transformative power of taking intentional steps to improve your sexual relationship, especially when your job as a first responder demands so much from you.

- **The importance of a healthy sex life in any relationship**

A healthy sex life is often considered one of the cornerstones of a fulfilling relationship. While sexual compatibility and satisfaction are not the only factors contributing to a relationship's longevity and quality, they play a pivotal role in emotional bonding, stress relief, and overall well-being. This section delves into the research and facts that emphasize why prioritizing a healthy sex life is crucial for any romantic relationship.

- **Emotional Bonding**

Sex is more than just a physical act; it's an intimate experience that fosters an emotional connection between partners. According to a study published in the Archives of Sexual Behavior, couples with a satisfying sex life tend to report higher levels of relationship satisfaction (Schoenfeld,

Loving, Pope, Huston, & Štulhofer, 2017). They found that 67% of couples who reported being sexually satisfied also reported confidence in their relationship.

- **Stress Relief**

Physical intimacy, including sexual activity, triggers the release of endorphins and other 'feel-good' hormones such as oxytocin. This hormone, often dubbed the 'cuddle hormone,' has been proven to reduce stress levels significantly. A study by the University of Zurich found that couples with frequent sexual intercourse had lower stress levels and better cognitive functions (Heiman, Long, Smith, Fisher, & Sand, 2011).

- **Health Benefits**

Regular sexual activity has been linked with various health benefits, from improved heart health to a more robust immune system. The American Heart Association notes that sexually active people have a 45% lower risk of developing heart diseases than those less active sexually. Moreover, sex burns about five calories per minute, making it an excellent (and enjoyable) form of exercise.

- **Satisfaction and Longevity in Relationships**

The National Opinion Research Center conducted a study revealing that couples with a satisfying sex life tend to stay together longer. Among those surveyed, 83% who reported having an active and fulfilling sexual relationship also stated they were less likely to consider divorce or separation than those who were sexually dissatisfied.

- **Cognitive and Psychological Effects**

Sexual activity and arousal stimulate brain function and have been linked to better cognitive abilities, including memory and problem-solving skills. A 2016 study by Coventry University in the U.K. revealed that people who have regular sexual activity scored higher on tests that measured their verbal fluency and ability to perceive objects and the spaces between them.

- **Self-Esteem and Relationship Quality**

Sexual satisfaction can significantly impact self-esteem and self-worth. According to a 2013 study published in the Journal of Social and Personal Relationships, people who are sexually satisfied in their relationships reported higher levels of self-esteem and were less likely to experience depression than those who are sexually unsatisfied.

Understanding how a healthy sex life can benefit you and your partner is the first step towards cultivating a fulfilling, lasting relationship. From emotional bonding and stress relief to numerous health benefits and relationship satisfaction, the role of a satisfying sexual relationship cannot be overstated.

Given the unique stressors first responders face, incorporating these findings into your relationship can act as a buffer against job-related emotional and physical strain, benefiting your romantic and professional life.

- **Specific challenges first responders face in maintaining a fulfilling sex life**

First responders face unique challenges that can adversely affect their personal lives, including their sexual relationships. The nature of their work—stressful, unpredictable, and often traumatic—can have profound implications for intimacy and sexual health. In this section, we'll discuss some key challenges specific to first responders and tackle frequently asked questions (FAQ) that may arise.

- **Irregular Work Hours**

First responders often work unpredictable shifts that can last for extended periods. This irregularity can disrupt sleep patterns and the opportunity for consistent intimate encounters with their partners.

FAQ:

Q: How can first responders manage time for intimacy amidst erratic work schedules?

A: *Scheduling "intimacy time" in advance and making the most available time are critical steps. Some couples find that syncing their digital calendars helps.*

- **Emotional and Psychological Stress**

The job involves high-stakes situations that can lead to emotional numbness or difficulty transitioning from a "work mode" to a more intimate mindset.

FAQ:

Q: What can be done to transition from work stress to being present in intimate moments?

A: *Implementing decompression routines, such as exercise or meditation, can help to shift gears mentally.*

- **Exposure to Traumatic Events**

Exposure to traumatic events can lead to conditions like PTSD, significantly affecting libido and emotional availability.

FAQ:

Q: Can therapy help maintain a sexual relationship while dealing with trauma?

A: *Yes, targeted therapies like cognitive behavioral therapy (CBT) have proven effective in helping people manage PTSD symptoms, including those affecting sexual health.*

- **Physical Exhaustion**

The job's physical demands can lead to fatigue, which may decrease sexual desire and performance.

FAQ:

Q: How can one manage physical fatigue and maintain an active sex life?

A: *Prioritizing sleep and regular exercise can improve energy levels and sexual performance.*

- **Risk of Occupational Hazards**

Exposure to harmful substances or environments may lead to health issues that affect sexual function.

FAQ:

Q: Are first responders at risk of sexual health issues due to occupational hazards?

A: *Though less common, risks do exist. Regular medical checks are crucial for monitoring any adverse effects on sexual or reproductive health.*

- **The 'Hero' Complex**

Being seen as a 'hero' can create unrealistic expectations, including in one's intimate relationships, potentially leading to performance anxiety.

FAQ:

Q: Does the societal image of a 'hero' affect first responders' sexual health?

A: *The pressure to 'perform' in all aspects of life, including the bedroom, can create stress and anxiety. It's important to communicate openly with your partner to manage these expectations.*

Understanding the unique challenges you may face as a first responder is the first step toward overcoming them. Open communication, professional help, and proactive management are vital in maintaining a fulfilling sexual relationship amidst these challenges.

THE IMPACT OF TRAUMATIC EVENTS ON A FIRST RESPONDER'S SEX DRIVE

Traumatic events can profoundly impact first responders' mental and emotional well-being, which may significantly affect their sexual health. The psychological toll of experiencing trauma can manifest in various ways, including reduced libido, sexual dysfunction, and difficulties in emotional intimacy. This section will explore how traumatic events can impact a first responder's sex drive and offer insights into managing this complex issue.

The Stress Response and Hormonal Imbalance

The body's natural response to stress involves the release of stress hormones like cortisol and adrenaline. While these hormones are vital for responding to emergencies, chronic exposure can lead to hormonal imbalances that may lower sexual desire.

PTSD and Libido

Post-Traumatic Stress Disorder (PTSD) is a common consequence of experiencing traumatic events and can significantly affect sexual desire. Studies have shown that individuals with PTSD are more likely to experience sexual dysfunction, including reduced libido, erectile dysfunction, or difficulties achieving orgasm.

Emotional Disconnection

Trauma can create an emotional barrier, making it difficult for first responders to connect emotionally with their partners. Emotional disconnection can lead to a decreased interest in sexual activity and may even cause aversion to physical intimacy.

Hyperarousal and Performance Anxiety

Hyperarousal is a common symptom of PTSD and can result in heightened stress responses, even in non-threatening situations. This heightened stress can translate to performance anxiety during sexual activity, making it challenging to maintain arousal and achieve sexual satisfaction.

Depersonalization and Derealization

Some individuals experience depersonalization (feeling disconnected from oneself) or derealization (feeling that the world is inaccurate) after trauma. These symptoms can make it challenging to engage in intimate relationships, both emotionally and sexually.

Coping Mechanisms and Risky Behavior

Some first responders may resort to risky sexual behavior as a coping mechanism after experiencing trauma. While this may provide temporary relief or distraction, it often exacerbates long-term problems within relationships and regarding personal health.

Therapeutic Interventions

Effective therapeutic interventions, like cognitive behavioral therapy (CBT) and Eye Movement Desensitization and Reprocessing (EMDR), can help individuals process trauma and restore emotional balance. In many cases, treating the underlying trauma can improve sexual health.

Traumatic experiences can significantly impact a first responder's sex drive, affecting their well-being and the health of their romantic relationships.

Understanding these challenges is the first step to managing them effectively, often requiring a multidisciplinary approach that may include psychological therapy, medical treatment, and open communication with one's partner. By addressing the root cause and seeking appropriate treatment, it's possible to restore a satisfying sex life while also improving overall emotional well-being.

The Role of Stress and Adrenaline

- Understanding the physical and mental toll of the job
- How stress affects libido and sexual performance
- Strategies to cope with work-induced stress

Stress and adrenaline are almost constant companions for first responders, always present at varying levels due to the demands and unpredictability of the job. While these physiological responses are essential for performance during high-pressure situations, they can also affect sexual health. Understanding the mechanisms and impact of stress and adrenaline on libido and sexual performance is crucial for maintaining a fulfilling romantic relationship.

- **Understanding the Physical and Mental Toll of the Job**

First responders are exposed to chronic stress, which puts them at risk for developing symptoms of burnout, depression, and anxiety. According to the Journal of Emergency Medical Services (JEMS), around 37% of first responders experience symptoms associated with Post-Traumatic Stress Disorder (PTSD). Such stress manifests mentally and physically, causing tension, fatigue, and, in some cases, hormonal imbalances, all of which can hamper sexual performance and desire.

- **How Stress Affects Libido and Sexual Performance**

Stress triggers the release of cortisol, a hormone that, when consistently high, can inhibit sexual arousal and performance. A study published in the Journal of Sexual Medicine found that men with high levels of workplace stress were 30% more likely to suffer from erectile dysfunction than those with lower stress levels. For women, high-stress levels can disrupt menstrual cycles and reduce sexual desire, as found in a 2015 study published in the Archives of Sexual Behavior.

- **Strategies to Cope with Work-induced Stress**

Mindfulness Meditation: Mindfulness techniques have been shown to reduce cortisol levels, improving both mental well-being and sexual performance.

Physical Exercise: Regular exercise boosts endorphin levels, countering the adverse effects of stress and improving libido. The American Heart Association suggests at least 150 minutes of moderate exercise per week for a balanced lifestyle.

Open Communication: Discussing work stress openly with a partner can build emotional support, improving sexual satisfaction.

Professional Help: Therapy and counseling services, especially those focusing on stress management, can provide long-term benefits for emotional and sexual well-being.

- **A Case Study: Anna and Mark**

Anna, an EMT, and Mark, a firefighter, have been married for five years. As they progressed in their careers, both noticed a significant dip in their sexual lives. The demanding hours and traumatic scenes each faced daily led to a cycle of stress and fatigue that stifled their intimacy.

Aware of the spiral they were in, they sought professional help. Mark started practicing mindfulness to manage his stress levels while Anna jogged to release endorphins. They also began attending couples therapy to build better communication strategies.

After six months, they both reported substantial improvements in their stress levels. Mirroring this change, their sexual lives also flourished. Anna's menstrual cycle became more regular, and both reported increased levels of sexual desire and satisfaction. The life of a first responder comes with unique stressors that can significantly impact one's sexual health. Understanding these physiological mechanisms and employing targeted coping strategies can mitigate the negative impacts of stress and adrenaline on both libido and performance.

COMMUNICATION IS KEY

- The need for open dialogue between partners
- Tips for effective communication about sex
- Choose the Right Time and Place: Select a moment when you are not distracted, stressed, or tired. The environment should be comfortable and private.
- Be Open and Honest: Honesty is critical in discussing sex. Be upfront about your desires, fears, and concerns.
- Use "I" Statements: Instead of saying, "You don't satisfy me," try saying, "I feel unsatisfied when we do this." This prevents your partner from feeling attacked and opens the door for constructive dialogue.

- Be Specific: General statements like "I'm not happy with our sex life" are not as helpful as specific comments like "I would enjoy our sexual encounters more if we could try XYZ."
- Listen Actively: Show genuine interest in your partner's thoughts and feelings. Make eye contact, nod, and don't interrupt.
- Avoid Blame: Criticism can make your counterproductive partner defensive. Focus on the issue, not the person.
- Be Positive and Affirmative: Compliment your partner on what they do right or what you enjoy, rather than focusing solely on what's wrong.
- Ask Open-Ended Questions: Instead of asking, "Do you like this?" ask, "How does this make you feel?" This opens the conversation and allows for more depth.
- Be Patient and Consistent: Resolving an issue may take multiple conversations. Please don't rush the process; let it develop naturally over time.
- Encourage Feedback: Make it clear that you value your partner's opinion and that the conversation is two-way.
- Be Receptive to Your Partner's Feelings: If your partner is opening up about something sensitive, acknowledge their courage and respond with understanding.
- Be Educated and Educate: If you're going to suggest trying something new, make sure you both know what it involves. Knowledge can lessen anxiety and enhance enjoyment.
- Be Mindful of Body Language: Sometimes, what's not said is as powerful as what is displayed. Pay attention to your partner's facial expressions, posture, and other nonverbal cues.
- Be Willing to Compromise: You may not agree on everything, and that's okay. What's important is finding a middle ground where both parties feel content and respected.

- Regular Check-Ins: Make it a habit to discuss your sexual health and happiness periodically. This keeps the lines of communication open and helps prevent minor issues from becoming major problems.

How lack of communication can lead to misunderstandings and dissatisfaction

- **Misaligned Expectations**

When partners do not communicate about their sexual preferences, needs, and boundaries, they operate on assumptions. These assumptions can lead to misaligned expectations where one partner may expect certain sexual activities that the other is uncomfortable with or unaware of.

- **Unresolved Issues and Resentment**

A lack of communication often means that big or small issues go unresolved. This could be as simple as preferences for certain sexual positions or as complex as addressing performance anxieties. Over time, these unresolved issues can build resentment, which can poison a relationship inside and outside the bedroom.

- **Emotional Distance**

Not talking about sex can create emotional barriers. When sexual needs are unmet or misunderstood, it can lead to feelings of rejection or inadequacy. This emotional distance can further reduce sexual desire, creating a vicious cycle of dissatisfaction.

- **Loss of Intimacy**

Poor communication can lead to decreased sexual activity and loss of intimacy. The less intimate moments a couple shares, the more they may feel disconnected, leading to a weakened emotional bond.

- **Lower Self-Esteem**

If either partner feels their sexual needs are not being met but cannot communicate this, it can decrease self-esteem. This can manifest in self-doubt and heightened insecurities, inhibiting open communication and sexual satisfaction.

- **Negative Impact on Overall Relationship Quality**

Poor communication in sexual matters can spill over into other areas of the relationship, affecting overall relationship quality. According to a study published in the Archives of Sexual Behavior, dissatisfaction in sexual life is strongly correlated with general discontent in a relationship.

- **Case Study: Sarah and Alex**

Sarah and Alex were together for two years, but their sex life had always been a bit of a taboo topic between them. Sarah was unhappy with their infrequent sexual encounters but never voiced her concerns, assuming Alex was satisfied with how things were. Alex retreated emotionally, Sensing Sarah's increasing detachment but not understanding the reason. After they finally decided to communicate their dissatisfaction openly, they realized that both had silently grappled with unmet sexual needs. They made an effort to prioritize open communication, which not only improved their sexual relationship but also enriched their emotional connection.

The lack of communication can profoundly impact relationships, leading to misunderstandings, unmet expectations, and dissatisfaction. The good news is that these problems are largely preventable through open, honest, and regular communication between partners.

QUIZ: ASSESSING COMMUNICATION AND SEXUAL SATISFACTION IN YOUR RELATIONSHIP

Instructions:

Select the answer that most closely aligns with your experience for each question. At the end of the quiz, tally your points to see where you stand on the communication and sexual satisfaction scale.

1. **How often do you and your partner discuss your sexual desires and preferences?**

   Never (1 point)

   Rarely (2 points)

   Sometimes (3 points)

   Often (4 points)

2. **Do you feel comfortable talking to your partner about sexual boundaries?**

   No, never (1 point)

   Sometimes, but it isn't easy (2 points)

   Mostly, yes (3 points)

   Absolutely (4 points)

3. **Have there been unresolved sexual issues between you and your partner?**

   Yes, many (1 point)

   A few (2 points)

   Not many (3 points)

   None (4 points)

4. **How often do you feel emotionally distant after a sexual encounter with your partner?**

   Always (1 point)

   Often (2 points)

   Rarely (3 points)

   Never (4 points)

5. **How would you rate your overall sexual satisfaction in your relationship?**

   Very dissatisfied (1 point)

   Somewhat disappointed (2 points)

   Satisfied (3 points)

   Very satisfied (4 points)

6. **Do you feel your sexual needs are met in your relationship?**

   No, not at all (1 point)

   Somewhat, but not entirely (2 points)

   Mostly, yes (3 points)

   Completely (4 points)

7. **Does poor sexual communication negatively impact other areas of your relationship?**

   Yes, frequently (1 point)

   Sometimes (2 points)

   Rarely (3 points)

   No, never (4 points)

8. **How confident do you feel about resolving sexual issues through communication?**

   Not confident at all (1 point)

   A little confident (2 points)

   Secure (3 points)

   Very confident (4 points)

Scoring:

8–16 Points: Your relationship may have significant communication and sexual satisfaction issues that need immediate attention. Consider seeking professional advice to address these concerns.

17–24 Points: While your relationship has some communication barriers concerning sexual matters, they are not insurmountable. Take steps to improve your communication and address your concerns openly.

25–28 Points: You have generally good communication and sexual satisfaction but should still strive for improvement. Open, honest conversations can constantly enrich a relationship.

29–32 Points: Congratulations! Your relationship excels in sexual communication and satisfaction. Continue your open dialogue to maintain this healthy aspect of your relationship.

This quiz will be a starting point for understanding how lack of communication can affect sexual satisfaction in your relationship. Consider speaking with a healthcare provider or a qualified relationship counselor for a more comprehensive understanding.

THE ROLE OF EMOTIONAL INTIMACY

- **The connection between emotional and sexual intimacy**

The connection between emotional and sexual intimacy in a relationship is intricate and deeply interwoven as mutually reinforcing pillars of a strong partnership. Emotional intimacy—trust, open communication, and emotional safety—often lays the groundwork for a fulfilling sexual relationship. Trust allows partners to explore their sexual boundaries freely. In contrast, open communication about desires and concerns leads to greater sexual satisfaction. Conversely, a healthy sexual relationship can enhance emotional intimacy by creating shared moments of vulnerability and closeness.

Research, such as studies published in the "Journal of Marriage and Family," substantiates this by indicating that trust and emotional intimacy are significant predictors of sexual satisfaction. Thus, a deficit in emotional or sexual intimacy often affects the other, emphasizing the importance of nurturing for a thriving romantic relationship.

Expanding on this interconnectedness, emotional and sexual intimacy often act as feedback loops for each other. A deeper emotional connection can pave the way for more satisfying and explorative sexual experiences, strengthening the emotional bond. Meanwhile, fulfilling sexual encounters can heighten feelings of emotional closeness and trust, creating a virtuous cycle that benefits the overall relationship.

On the flip side, a lack of emotional intimacy can lead to sexual dissatisfaction due to insecurities or a lack of openness in discussing sexual needs, and an unsatisfying sexual life can exacerbate emotional distance or even breed resentment. Studies have also shown that couples with high levels of emotional intimacy often report higher levels of sexual satisfaction and vice versa. For example, research in the "Archives of Sexual Behavior" suggests that emotional intimacy is not only a predictor for sexual pleasure but also overall relationship satisfaction. Thus, the two are not isolated constructs but deeply interlinked facets of a relationship that jointly contribute to its health and longevity.

As of my last training data in September 2021, numerous studies have explored the interplay between emotional and sexual intimacy in relationships.

Here are a few:

Journal of Marriage and Family: Several studies published in this journal have demonstrated a strong correlation between trust, emotional intimacy, and sexual satisfaction. One study indicated that couples who reported higher levels of trust also reported greater satisfaction in their sexual lives.

Archives of Sexual Behavior: This journal has published research suggesting that emotional intimacy is not only a significant predictor of sexual satisfaction but also overall relationship satisfaction.

Journal of Sex & Marital Therapy: Studies in this journal have delved into the nuances between emotional intimacy and sexual satisfaction, indicating that effective communication about sexual needs and preferences leads to a more satisfying sexual relationship, enhancing emotional intimacy.

Social Psychological and Personality Science: This journal has published work suggesting that sexual satisfaction can predict future levels of commitment and emotional satisfaction, providing evidence for the cyclical nature of emotional and sexual intimacy.

Health Psychology: Studies here have examined how chronic stress and emotional well-being impact sexual satisfaction, underlining the importance of emotional health for a satisfying sexual life.

Psychology of Men & Masculinity: Research focusing on men's emotional and sexual well-being indicates that emotional intimacy is critical for men's sexual satisfaction, contradicting stereotypes that men are only interested in the physical aspects of sex.

These studies offer compelling evidence for the strong connection between emotional and sexual intimacy, each amplifying and enhancing the other in a loop that contributes significantly to the overall health of a relationship. It would be advisable to consult academic databases and peer-reviewed journals for the most current research.

- **Navigating emotional numbness or PTSD**

Emotional numbness and Post-Traumatic Stress Disorder (PTSD) can significantly affect one's sexual life, often resulting in diminished libido, intimacy issues, and even avoidance of sexual contact. Understanding how these psychological conditions interact with sexual intimacy is vital for treatment and healing.

THE COMPLEX INTERPLAY

Impact on Libido: Emotional numbness and PTSD can lead to a reduction in sexual drive. According to a study in the "Journal of Sexual Medicine," approximately 31% of individuals with PTSD reported sexual dysfunction.

Avoidance Behavior: A heightened state of emotional sensitivity or numbness can lead to avoidance of sexual intimacy as a coping mechanism.

Dissociation During Intimacy: Emotional numbness can lead to dissociative experiences during sexual activities, impacting the quality of the intimate connection.

COMMON CHALLENGES AND FAQ

Q: Can PTSD therapy improve my sexual life?

A: *Trauma-focused therapy can help address underlying issues that impact sexual function and intimacy.*

Q: How do I discuss my emotional numbness with my partner without making them feel inadequate?

A: *Open and honest communication is crucial. Assure your partner that emotional numbness is a symptom of your condition, not a reflection of your feelings towards them.*

Q: Can medication for PTSD affect sexual function?

A: *Yes, medications like SSRIs can have sexual side effects. Consult with a healthcare provider for tailored advice.*

Strategies for Coping
- Seek Professional Help: Individual and couples therapy can provide effective coping mechanisms.
- Mindfulness Techniques: Mindfulness can help reconnect with one's body and sensations, which can benefit sexual intimacy.
- Open Communication: Partners should aim for a safe space where both can express their feelings and concerns openly.

CASE STORY: EMILY AND MARK

A combat veteran, Emily struggled with PTSD, affecting her relationship with Mark, particularly their sexual life. After seeking trauma-focused therapy, Emily learned coping strategies that helped her re-engage in intimate moments without triggering her PTSD symptoms. As she healed, their emotional and sexual intimacy improved, reinforcing each other positively. While emotional numbness and PTSD challenge sexual intimacy, they are not insurmountable. A multi-faceted approach that includes professional guidance, open communication, and individual coping strategies can help couples navigate these complex issues and maintain a fulfilling sexual relationship.

Creating a safe space for emotional connection is essential for fostering both emotional and sexual intimacy in a relationship. In a non-judgmental and open environment, partners are more likely to express their desires, fears, and concerns without fearing rejection or ridicule. This openness often translates into a more fulfilling sexual relationship, as trust and communication are cornerstones of sexual satisfaction. A safe emotional space doesn't just enable dialogue; it enhances the quality of the intimacy experienced by both partners, allowing them to explore their sexual boundaries and preferences in a secure, trusting atmosphere.

> *The idea of creating a safe space for emotional and sexual intimacy within a relationship; Ephesians 4:32:*
>
> *"Be kind to one another, tenderhearted, forgiving one another, as God in Christ forgave you."*

This verse emphasizes the importance of kindness, compassion, and forgiveness, critical components for creating a safe emotional space. These attributes can go a long way in establishing the trust and open communication essential for deep emotional and sexual intimacy in a relationship.

PHYSICAL HEALTH AND ITS IMPACT

Maintaining physical well-being is intrinsically linked to sexual health, with numerous studies indicating that exercise and a balanced diet can significantly enhance sexual function and satisfaction. For instance, according to the "Journal of Sexual Medicine," regular aerobic exercise can improve erectile function and overall sexual performance. Furthermore, periodic medical check-ups are crucial in monitoring sexual health; screenings for STIs, hormonal imbalances, and other health issues can preemptively address potential obstacles to a fulfilling sex life.

Alongside this, healthy habits like reducing alcohol consumption and quitting smoking can notably improve sexual function. A 2015 study in the "American Journal of Men's Health" revealed that smokers are more likely to suffer from erectile dysfunction than non-smokers. For those facing sexual health issues, treatments range from medications and hormone therapy to lifestyle changes and counseling. The key is to proactively manage your physical health as a gateway to improving your sexual life.

The intricate relationship between physical well-being and sexual health is an area that can't be overstated. Physical fitness boosts self-esteem and enhances blood flow and hormonal balance, directly impacting sexual function. For example, a study published in "Obesity" found that weight loss significantly improved sexual satisfaction. Regular medical check-ups, including prostate exams for men and pelvic exams for women, can catch issues like erectile dysfunction, vaginal dryness, or low libido early on, making treatment more effective. Regular screenings for conditions like high blood pressure or diabetes, which can adversely affect sexual health, are also recommended.

Dietary habits also play an undeniable role; foods rich in antioxidants and omega-3 fatty acids have been linked to better sexual function. Abstinence from detrimental habits like excessive drinking is also crucial, as alcohol can depress sexual performance. As for healing and improvement, consult healthcare providers for tailored treatment plans, including medication, hormone replacement therapy, or psychosexual counseling for both partners. Natural remedies and exercises, such as Kegel exercises for pelvic floor strengthening, can also be helpful. A comprehensive, proactive approach to physical health is one of the most effective strategies for enhancing sexual wellness.

PSYCHOLOGICAL BARRIERS

Beyond the Bedroom: Cultivating Intimacy Outside of Sexual Activities and Maintaining Connection During Periods of Sexual Inactivity

While sexual intimacy is essential to romantic relationships, it's not the sole form of closeness between partners. Familiarity extends beyond the bedroom, and maintaining a connection during periods of sexual inactivity is crucial for the overall health of the relationship.

This section explores the various ways to foster emotional closeness and the significance of non-sexual forms of intimacy.

INTIMACY OUTSIDE OF SEXUAL ACTIVITIES

Emotional Connection: One of the most essential forms of intimacy, emotional closeness involves open communication, trust, and a shared sense of purpose.

Intellectual Intimacy: Being on the same page intellectually allows couples to engage in stimulating conversations and shared learning experiences, leading to a deeper emotional connection.

Experiential Intimacy: Engaging in shared activities or hobbies can be another powerful way to deepen intimacy. Whether cooking together, taking a dance class, or hiking, shared experiences create a sense of partnership and mutual growth.

MAINTAINING CONNECTION DURING PERIODS OF SEXUAL INACTIVITY

Open Communication: During sexual inactivity, whether due to medical reasons, stress, or other life events, keeping the lines of communication open is essential. Discuss your feelings and concerns and ensure you understand the reason behind the temporary hiatus.

Physical Touch: Even if you're not engaging in sexual activities, other forms of physical touch, like hugs, kisses, and cuddling, can maintain a sense of physical closeness.

Quality Time: Spend quality time together doing activities that you both enjoy. This nurtures the emotional component of your relationship, maintaining a connection despite sexual inactivity.

Revisiting Memories: Go through old photos, reminisce about shared experiences, or revisit where you first met to rekindle the emotional intimacy.

Intimacy is multifaceted and extends well beyond sexual activities. Especially during periods when sexual activity may be reduced or absent, focusing on other forms of intimacy is essential to keep the relationship strong. Emotional closeness, intellectual connection, and shared experiences can provide a rich tapestry of intimacy that enhances the relationship in different yet equally significant ways.

In a small town where everyone knew each other's names, Officers Jane and Mark had been partners on the force for several years. Both had seen their fair share of life's darker moments, which brought a depth of understanding to their professional relationship. They realized their bond extended beyond the badge and duty as time passed. During a period when their demanding schedules and traumatic experiences led to a hiatus in their sexual intimacy, they made a conscious effort to maintain their emotional connection.

One evening, after a grueling shift, they decided to revisit the lakeside park, where they first realized their feelings for each other. As they sat on the bench, looking at the moonlit water, they held hands and began to share their thoughts and fears openly, discussing the recent emotional toll of their work. This heartfelt conversation became a turning point in their relationship. Although they couldn't immediately resolve all the stress and trauma affecting their sexual intimacy, this moment of emotional connection fortified their relationship. Both felt a renewed sense of closeness, reminding them that intimacy was not confined to the physical but deeply rooted in emotional and experiential bonds.

PRACTICAL TIPS AND RESOURCES
Mobile Apps for Tracking Sexual Health
Clue: Primarily aimed at tracking menstrual cycles, Clue also offers insights into how different process phases can affect libido.

MyMoxie: A sexual wellness app designed to educate users on various aspects of sexual health, including common sexual dysfunctions and remedies.

Sexual Health Guide: Offers information on STIs, contraceptive methods, and general sexual health advice.

RECOMMENDED READING AND TOOLS
Come As You Are **by Emily Nagoski:** A comprehensive look into the science of female sexuality, breaking down cultural myths and offering actionable advice.

The 5 Love Languages **by Gary Chapman:** While not strictly about sexual health, understanding your love language can significantly improve your emotional and sexual connection. I have read this, and it's very recommended.

We-Vibe Sync: A couple's vibrator designed to enhance physical intimacy, improving the sexual experience for both partners.

EXPERT ADVICE AND RECOMMENDED PROFESSIONALS

Certified Sex Therapists (CST): These are therapists trained explicitly in addressing sexual issues and can be invaluable for couples or individuals experiencing challenges.

Urologists and Gynecologists: For physiological issues affecting sexual health, these specialists can offer both diagnoses and treatments.

Psychiatrists/Psychologists specializing in PTSD or Emotional Numbness: Given first responders' unique challenges, consulting professionals in this area can benefit those dealing with emotional trauma affecting their sexual life.

Improving and maintaining your sexual health is a multifaceted endeavor that benefits from various resources. Mobile apps can offer real-time tracking and insights, while a well-chosen reading list and valuable tools can provide knowledge and actionable solutions. Finally, don't underestimate the value of expert consultations for personalized, effective treatments and strategies. Whether facing emotional obstacles or seeking to improve a healthy sexual relationship, these resources can provide invaluable support.

CHAPTER CONCLUSION

Maintaining a healthy sex life is especially crucial for first responders, given the job's high-stress and emotionally demanding nature. Sexual intimacy serves not just as a physical release but also as an emotional refuge, a place where the barriers can come down, and authentic connection can occur. It becomes a sanctuary of mutual trust, emotional vulnerability, and relaxation, attributes often missing from the daily grind of a first responder's routine.

The ongoing journey of maintaining sexual health in a high-stress occupation is not a destination but a continual process. It involves a blend of emotional, physical, and psychological attentiveness, which resources such as mobile apps, recommended reading, and professional consultations can aid. Despite the challenges, the endeavor is worthwhile for the overall well-being of the individual and the relationship. Investing in a fulfilling sexual life is not just beneficial but imperative for first responders, a key element in a holistic approach to managing the rigors of a taxing yet vital profession.

CHAPTER 4

Balancing Work and Personal Life

One of the biggest challenges of being a first responder is balancing work and personal life. This chapter will discuss ways to manage work-life balance, including setting boundaries and prioritizing quality time with loved ones.

Balancing work and personal life can significantly challenge first responders, substantially impacting their relationships. This chapter will discuss the importance of finding a healthy balance between work and personal life and provide strategies.

Understanding the Importance of Work-Life Balance: First responders and their partners must realize the importance of balancing work and personal life. This balance is essential for maintaining physical, mental, and emotional well-being and can help to strengthen the relationship.

Setting Priorities: First responders and their partners must set priorities to ensure that they can find a healthy balance between work and personal life. This includes setting aside time for work-related and individual activities, such as spending time with family and friends.

Planning can help first responders and their partners find a healthy balance between work and personal life. This can include scheduling regular time off from work, planning family activities, and setting aside time for self-care.

Establishing Boundaries: Clear boundaries between work and personal life can help first responders and their partners find a healthy balance. This includes setting limits on work-related activities at home, avoiding work-related phone calls during personal time, and disconnecting from work when at home.

Setting boundaries is essential to maintaining a healthy relationship, especially for first responders and partners facing unique trauma exposure and shift work challenges.

Here are some ways to set boundaries:
Communicate your needs, feelings, and boundaries to your partner. This will help to establish a mutual understanding and respect for each other's boundaries.

Set limits on work talk: Establish limits on how much work-related speech you will engage in at home. This helps create a healthy balance between work and personal life.

Prioritize self-care: Set aside time for self-care activities, such as exercise, meditation, or hobbies, and prioritize this time as sacred.

Create designated "off" times: Designate specific times during the day or week when you will be "off" from work and communicate this to your partner and colleagues.

Maintain physical and emotional space: Respect each other's physical and emotional freedom by avoiding intrusive behavior and respecting privacy.

Establish technology boundaries: Establish boundaries around technology use, such as not using phones or computers during certain times or in specific spaces, like the bedroom.

Seek professional help: If necessary, seek professional help to address boundary-related issues and learn additional strategies for setting and maintaining healthy boundaries.

Setting boundaries is crucial to maintaining a healthy relationship, and establishing and supporting them takes effort and intentional action. Remember, boundaries are not meant to restrict or limit your relationship but to create a healthy and supportive environment for both partners.

Encouraging Self-Care: Self-care, such as regular exercise, a healthy diet, and enough sleep, can help first responders and their partners find a healthy balance between work and personal life. Self-care is essential for maintaining physical, mental, and emotional well-being and can help to strengthen relationships by reducing stress and improving overall health. Engaging in shared self-care activities, such as cooking healthy meals or going for walks, can create a strong bond and provide opportunities for quality time together.

Incorporating self-care into your daily routine can take effort, but the benefits are well worth it. Some self-care activities that can be helpful include:

Exercise: Regular physical activity, such as running, yoga, or weightlifting, can help to reduce stress, improve mood, and maintain physical health.

Relaxation techniques: Engaging in relaxation techniques, such as deep breathing, meditation, or massage, can help to reduce stress and improve overall well-being.

Healthy diet: Eating a balanced diet with plenty of fruits, vegetables, and whole grains can help maintain physical health and improve mood.

Adequate sleep: Getting enough sleep, at least 7-9 hours per night, is essential for physical and mental health.

Hobbies and interests: Engaging in hobbies and interests, such as reading, playing music, or gardening, can provide an outlet for stress and improve overall well-being.

Remember, self-care is not selfish. It is essential. Encouraging and prioritizing self-care can help first responders and their partners maintain their health and well-being, which in turn can strengthen their relationship.

Seeking Support: Seeking support from family, friends, or a support group that can help first responders and their partners find a healthy balance between work and personal life. This support can provide additional resources and support during difficult times and can help to strengthen the relationship.

Being Available for Each Other: First responders and their partners must be available for each other to ensure that they can find a healthy balance between work and personal life. This can include scheduling regular date nights, taking trips, or simply spending quality time together. Being available for each other is essential to any relationship, especially for first responders and their partners who face unique trauma exposure and shift work challenges. Availability refers to being physically, emotionally, and mentally present to your partner. This means being open and receptive to their needs, feelings, and experiences and being willing to offer support and understanding.

One way to be available is by setting aside dedicated time for each other, such as regular date nights or weekend getaways. This time can be used to catch up on each other's lives, share experiences, and enjoy each other's company. Additionally, listening actively and responding empathetically to each other's concerns can foster a sense of closeness and understanding.

It is also essential to recognize that being available for each other may involve making sacrifices, such as adjusting schedules or priorities, to be present for your partner. This can include supporting each other during difficult times, such as during a deployment or after a traumatic call, or simply being there for each other during everyday life events. Being available for each other is not always easy, but it is essential to maintaining a healthy relationship. By trying to be present for each other and offer support, first responders and their partners can strengthen their bond and create a supportive environment for each other.

Practicing Flexibility: Flexibility can help first responders and their partners find a healthy balance between work and personal life. This includes being open to schedule changes, adjusting priorities, and understanding each other's needs. Flexibility is essential to maintaining a healthy relationship, especially for first responders and partners facing unique trauma exposure-related challenges, shift work, and unpredictable schedules. Flexibility refers to the ability to adapt to changing circumstances and adjust to new situations as they arise.

In a relationship, flexibility involves being open to different perspectives and willing to compromise when necessary. This can include changing your routine or schedule to accommodate each other's needs, being willing to try new activities and experiences, and being open to constructive feedback and suggestions. Flexibility also involves adapting to unique circumstances and unexpected events, such as work schedule changes or deployment. This can mean being willing to adjust plans or make sacrifices to support each other during difficult times. It is essential to recognize that practicing flexibility requires effort and a willingness to compromise.

However, by being flexible and open-minded, first responders and their partners can create a supportive and understanding environment for each other. This, in turn, can help to strengthen the relationship and improve overall well-being.

TAKING TIME FOR PERSONAL INTERESTS

First responders and their partners must take time for personal interests to find a healthy balance between work and personal life. This can include pursuing hobbies, volunteering, or engaging in leisure activities. Taking time for personal interests is essential to self-care and maintaining a healthy relationship, especially for first responders and their partners who face unique challenges related to trauma exposure, shift work, and stress. Personal interests refer to activities and hobbies that bring joy, fulfillment, and a sense of purpose outside your relationship.

Personal interests and passions can reduce stress and improve overall well-being. It can also provide a sense of identity and independence, which can be crucial in maintaining a healthy relationship. When taking time for personal interests, it is vital to communicate with your partner and find a balance that works for both of you. This may involve scheduling time for individual pursuits, such as hobbies or exercise, or finding shared interests to enjoy together.

It is also essential to recognize that personal interests may change over time, which is okay. Encouraging and supporting each other's interests can create a supportive and understanding environment, ultimately strengthening the relationship.

FINDING A SUPPORTIVE WORK ENVIRONMENT

Finding a supportive work environment, such as a workplace that values work-life balance, can help first responders and their partners find a healthy balance between work and personal life. A supportive work environment can provide additional resources and support to help first responders manage the job's demands. Finding a supportive work environment is essential for first responders and their partners who face unique challenges related to trauma exposure, shift work, and stress. A supportive work environment refers to a workplace that values and prioritizes the well-being of its employees and provides resources and support for coping with the challenges of the job. A supportive work environment can help reduce stress, improve mental and physical health, and increase job satisfaction. This can include having access to resources such as mental health support, flexible schedules, and opportunities for professional growth.

First responders and their partners must communicate with their employers and advocate for their needs. This may involve seeking out resources, such as an Employee Assistance Program, or having open and honest conversations with supervisors and colleagues about the challenges of the job and the importance of self-care. Having a supportive work environment can also have a positive impact on relationships. A supportive workplace can reduce stress and increase job satisfaction, improving well-being and strengthening relationships.

MAKING FLEXIBILITY A PRIORITY

Making flexibility a priority in work and personal life can help first responders and their partners find a healthy balance. This includes being open to schedule changes, adjusting preferences, and understanding each other's needs. Making flexibility a focus is crucial for first responders and their partners who face unique challenges related to trauma exposure, shift work, and stress. Flexibility refers to adapting and adjusting to changes in circumstances, schedules, and priorities.

Flexibility can help reduce stress and improve overall well-being in a relationship by allowing both partners to prioritize their individual needs and the relationship's needs. This can include adjusting schedules to accommodate shift work, making time for self-care, and being open to change.

It is also essential to recognize that flexibility is a two-way street, and both partners should try to accommodate each other's needs. This can involve being understanding and supportive when plans change and finding ways to work together to find a solution that works for both of you.

ENCOURAGING WORK-LIFE INTEGRATION

Encouraging work-life integration, where work and personal life are integrated rather than separated, can help first responders and their partners to find a healthy balance. This can include finding ways to incorporate personal interests into work and bringing work-related skills and knowledge into private life. Work-life integration can also involve finding ways to make the most of time spent together, such as incorporating shared hobbies and interests into daily life. This can strengthen the relationship and create a shared purpose and fulfillment.

Encouraging work-life integration can also involve supporting each other's careers and personal growth. This can include encouraging each other to pursue education or training opportunities and finding ways to support each other's professional goals.

It is essential to recognize that work-life integration can look different for each person and each relationship and that what works for one couple may not work for another. It is crucial to have open and honest conversations about what work-life integration means for each person and to find a balance that works for both partners.

FOSTERING A POSITIVE WORK CULTURE

Fostering a positive work culture, where work-life balance is valued and encouraged, can help first responders and their partners find a healthy balance. A positive work culture can provide additional resources and support to help first responders manage the job's demands. A positive work culture can also help reduce stress and increase job satisfaction, improving first responders' well-being. This can include providing resources for self-care, offering flexible schedules, and encouraging open communication between management and staff. In a positive work culture, first responders are also more likely to feel supported and valued, which can help to reduce feelings of isolation and improve overall well-being. This can also lead to improved job performance, as first responders who feel supported and valued are more likely to be engaged and committed to their work.

For partners of first responders, a positive work culture can provide additional support and resources, such as access to counseling services, support groups, and educational resources. This can help partners better understand and manage the effects of trauma exposure and shift work on their relationship.

SEEKING ACCOMMODATIONS

First responders and their partners may benefit from seeking accommodation, such as flexible schedules or telecommuting, to help them find a healthy balance between work and personal life. Accommodation can provide additional resources and support to help first responders manage the job's demands. Concession can help first responders reduce the job's physical and emotional needs. This can help to reduce stress and improve overall well-being. For example, having a flexible schedule can give first responders more time for self-care and personal interests, leading to a better work-life balance.

There are several ways for first responders and their partners to seek accommodations to help them find a healthy balance between work and personal life.

These include:

Talking to your employer: First responders and their partners should have an open and honest conversation with their employer about their needs and the accommodations they require.

This can include flexible schedules, telecommuting, or modified duties.

Seeking support from a union or professional association: First responders who are members of a merger or professional association can seek help and advocacy from these organizations in seeking accommodations.

Utilizing available resources: First responders and their partners can use resources like employee assistance programs (EAPs) or human resources departments to seek accommodations.

Negotiating with your employer: First responders and their partners can negotiate to find a solution that works for both parties. This may involve compromising hours or duties, but it can help find a solution that works for both parties.

Seeking legal support: In some cases, first responders and their partners may need legal aid to protect their rights and receive the accommodations they need.

There are several ways for first responders and their partners to seek accommodations to help them find a healthy balance between work and personal life. By talking to their employer, seeking support from a union or professional association, utilizing available resources, negotiating with their employer, or seeking legal help, first responders and their partners can find the accommodations they need to improve their overall well-being and relationships.

For partners of first responders, accommodations such as telecommuting can provide additional support and resources, such as access to counseling services, support groups, and educational resources. This can help partners better understand and manage the effects of trauma exposure and shift work on their relationship.

ENCOURAGING FAMILY INVOLVEMENT

Encouraging family involvement in work-related activities, such as attending events or volunteering, can help first responders and their partners find a healthy balance between work and personal life. Family involvement can provide additional resources and support to help first responders manage the demands of the job and can also help to strengthen the relationship.

Encouraging family involvement in a first responder's association can enhance the bond between partners and create a supportive network. Some ways to promote family involvement include inviting family members to participate in joint activities, such as vacations, picnics, or game nights; encouraging open communication between family members, where feelings and experiences can be shared in a safe and supportive environment; and including family members in decision-making, such as when making plans or discussing future goals.

Such associations encourage family members to be involved in the first responder's recovery process, such as through counseling or support groups. They help to build a solid support network where family members can provide additional resources and support to help the first responder manage the job's demands. By involving family members in the relationship, first responders and their partners can create a supportive network that can help to improve their overall well-being and strengthen the bond between partners.

MAKING TIME FOR SELF-REFLECTION

Making time for self-reflection, such as journaling or meditating, can help first responders and their partners find a healthy balance between work and personal life. Self-reflection can provide insight into personal priorities and values and help ensure that work and personal life are aligned. Making time for self-reflection is critical to maintaining a healthy first-responder relationship.

Some ways to encourage self-reflection include:
- Setting aside dedicated time for self-reflection, such as through journaling or meditating
- Encouraging open communication, where feelings and experiences can be shared in a safe and supportive environment.
- Seeking support from a mental health professional, such as a therapist or counselor.

They are engaging in mindfulness practices, such as deep breathing exercises or mindful movement, Building a solid support system where friends, family, and community can provide additional resources and support. First responders and their partners can better understand their thoughts, feelings, and experiences and can work towards improving their overall well-being and relationships.

ENCOURAGING TEAM BUILDING

Encouraging team-building activities, such as retreats or teambuilding exercises, can help first responders and their partners find a healthy balance between work and personal life. Team building activities can provide additional resources and support to help first responders manage the demands of the job and can also help to strengthen the relationship.

Team building activities can help first responders build strong relationships with their colleagues and foster a positive work culture. Some tips for encouraging team building include:

- Encourage first responders to share their thoughts, feelings, and experiences with their colleagues. This helps build trust and increase understanding between team members.

- Plan fun and interactive activities like team-building exercises, group outings, or games. These activities can build camaraderie and improve team morale.
- Encourage first responders to collaborate on projects and assignments. This can build trust, increase understanding, and improve teamwork skills. Encourage healthy competition among team members, such as friendly sports games or challenges. This can create a sense of community and enhance team morale.
- Provide opportunities for personal growth for first responders to develop their skills and knowledge, such as training programs or workshops. This can help to improve job performance and increase job satisfaction. Celebrate the team's successes and acknowledge individual team members' hard work and dedication. This can build a positive work culture and improve team morale.
- Team building activities are essential to building strong relationships and fostering a positive work culture for first responders. By encouraging open communication, planning fun activities, and promoting healthy competition, first responders can build strong relationships with their colleagues and improve overall well-being.

FOSTERING A POSITIVE HOME LIFE

Fostering a positive home life, where family and personal life are valued and encouraged, can help first responders and their partners find a healthy balance between work and personal life. Positive home life can provide additional resources and support to help first responders manage the demands of the job and can also help to strengthen the relationship.

Fostering a positive home life is vital for maintaining a healthy first-responder relationship. Some ways to encourage a positive home life include:

- Encouraging open communication and emotional expression, where feelings and experiences can be shared in a safe and supportive environment.
- Building a solid support system where friends, family, and community can provide additional resources and support.
- Engaging in shared hobbies and interests, such as cooking, gardening, or playing sports together
- Practicing gratitude and celebrating successes, big or small
- Finding healthy coping mechanisms, such as physical activity or creative expression, to manage the effects of trauma exposure
- Making self-care a priority, including regular exercise, a healthy diet, and enough sleep
- Seeking professional help, if necessary, to manage the effects of trauma exposure
- Fostering a positive home life, first responders and their partners can build stronger relationships and improve overall well-being.

ENCOURAGING PROFESSIONAL DEVELOPMENT

sProfessional development, such as continuing education or skill-building workshops, can help first responders and their partners find a healthy balance between work and personal life. Professional development can provide additional resources and support to help. Encouraging professional development is a vital aspect of supporting first responders' well-being and career growth.

Some tips for encouraging professional development include:
Providing opportunities for training and education: Provide first responders with opportunities for training and education, such as workshops, conferences, or online courses. This can help to improve job performance and increase job satisfaction.

Encouraging goal setting: Encourage first responders to set professional and personal goals and support achieving those goals. This can help to improve job performance and increase job satisfaction.

Offering mentorship programs: Offer mentorship programs to help first responders connect with experienced professionals who can provide guidance and support.

Encouraging networking: Encourage first responders to network with other professionals in their field, such as attending conferences or joining professional organizations. This can help to improve job performance and increase job satisfaction.

Providing opportunities for advancement: For first responders to advance their careers, such as promotions or leadership positions. This can help to improve job performance and increase job satisfaction.

Recognizing achievements: Recognize the accomplishments of first responders, such as promotions or certifications, and celebrate their successes. This can help to improve job performance and increase job satisfaction.

Encouraging professional development is vital to supporting first responders' well-being and career growth. First responders can improve their job performance and increase job satisfaction by providing opportunities for training and education, motivating goal setting, and offering mentorship programs.

MAINTAINING A POSITIVE ATTITUDE

A positive attitude, even during difficult times, can help first responders and their partners find a healthy balance between work and personal life. A cheerful outlook can help to reduce stress and improve overall well-being.

What to do if your spouse is opposing all the time . . .

Managing a positive attitude when your spouse is opposing can be challenging, but it is possible. Here are some tips to help you maintain a positive attitude in these circumstances:

Practice self-care: Taking care of yourself physically and emotionally can help you maintain a positive outlook. This includes exercise, mindfulness, and engaging in hobbies you enjoy.

Establish healthy boundaries: Set clear boundaries with your spouse about what behaviors you will and will not tolerate. This can help you maintain a positive outlook and protect yourself from negativity.

Communicate openly and honestly: Open and honest communication is critical to maintaining a positive attitude. Share your feelings and concerns with your spouse and listen to their perspective.

Focus on the positives: When your spouse opposes, focus on the positive aspects of your relationship and life. This can help you maintain a positive outlook.

Seek outside support: Contact a trusted friend, family member, or therapist. They can provide a fresh perspective and help you manage your emotions.

Practicing gratitude can help you maintain a positive outlook, even in difficult circumstances. Take time each day to reflect on the things you are thankful for.

Seek professional help: If negativity affects your well-being, consider seeking a mental health professional. They can provide guidance and support for managing negative emotions and maintaining a positive attitude. It is crucial to prioritize your well-being and happiness. With time and effort, you can maintain a positive attitude and build a healthy relationship with your spouse.

ENCOURAGING OPEN COMMUNICATION

Encouraging open communication, where both partners feel comfortable sharing their thoughts and feelings, can help first responders and their partners find a healthy balance between work and personal life. Open communication can provide additional resources and support to help first responders manage the demands of the job and can also help to strengthen the relationship. Open communication is crucial to building healthy relationships, whether in personal or professional settings.

Here are some tips for promoting open communication:
Create a Safe Environment: Creating a safe and non-judgmental space for people to share their thoughts and ideas is essential. This can be achieved by listening, being empathetic, and avoiding adverse reactions or criticism.

Be an Active Listener: Listening to others when speaking actively is essential. This means paying attention to what they are saying, asking clarifying questions, and reflecting on what you have heard to ensure understanding.

Use Open-Ended Questions: Asking open-ended questions encourages people to share more about themselves and their thoughts. This helps create a more natural and open conversation.

Be Transparent: Encourage transparency by being open and honest in your communication. This can build trust and encourage others to do the same.

Respect Differences: Everyone has different opinions, beliefs, and backgrounds. Respecting these differences and approaching communication openly and without judgment is essential.

Provide Feedback: Feedback is a vital component of open communication. It is important to provide constructive feedback non-judgmentally to help people improve and grow.

Practice Active Communication: Encourage people to speak up and actively engage in conversations. This can promote a culture of open communication and lead to better decision-making and problem-solving.

Promoting open communication requires creating a safe environment, being an active listener, using open-ended questions, being transparent, respecting differences, providing feedback, and practicing active communication. These tips can encourage open communication and build healthy relationships in any setting.

SEEKING SUPPORT FROM COLLEAGUES

Seeking support from colleagues can help first responders and their partners find a healthy balance between work and personal life. Colleagues can provide additional resources and support to help first responders manage the demands of the job and can also help to strengthen the relationship.

Making Time for Fun: Making fun, such as participating in leisure activities or taking trips, can help first responders and their partners find a healthy balance between work and personal life. Having fun can provide a much-needed break from work demands and can help strengthen the relationship.

Building a Strong Support System: Building a solid support system, which includes family, friends, and community members, can help first responders and their partners find a healthy balance between work and personal life. A robust support system can provide additional resources and support during difficult times and can help to strengthen the relationship. A powerful support system can be crucial for our overall well-being and success.

Here are some tips for building a solid support system:
Identify your needs: Think about the areas where you need support. Do you need emotional support, help with practical tasks, or advice and guidance? Knowing what you need can help you identify the right people to turn to for support.

Reach out to friends and family: Do not be afraid to ask for help and support from the people closest to you. Share your feelings and concerns with them and tell them how they can help.

Join a community: Joining groups and communities can be a great way to meet new people who share your interests and values. Whether it is a local sports team, a hobby group, or a volunteer organization, being part of a community can provide a sense of belonging and support.

Seek professional help: Sometimes, we need more than just the support of our friends and family. Seeking professional help from a therapist, counselor, or coach can give us the tools and guidance to navigate difficult situations and build a more robust support system.

Be a good friend: Building solid relationships requires effort on both sides. Be there for your friends and family when they need support, and offer help and guidance when possible. By being a good friend, you will attract the same kind of support in return.

Remember, building a solid support system takes time and effort. But with persistence and a willingness to reach out to others, you can create a network of people who will be there for you through the ups and downs of life.

QUIZ TIME:

Here is a quiz you can take to see how positive you are:

When faced with a challenging situation, do you:
- A) Focus on the negative aspects of the situation.
- B) Find ways to turn the situation into a positive.

When you think about your future, do you:
- A) Worry about what could go wrong?
- B) Focus on the possibilities and opportunities.

When you make a mistake, do you:
- A) Beat yourself up about it?
- B) Learn from the experience and move forward.

When someone compliments you, do you:
- A) Dismiss the compliment?
- B) Accept the compliment with gratitude?

When you compare yourself to others, do you:
- A) Focus on what you lack.
- B) Celebrate your unique qualities and strengths.

When things do not go as planned, do you:
- A) Get upset and dwell on what went wrong.
- B) Look for opportunities to learn and grow.

When faced with a difficult decision, do you:

A) Focus on the risks and adverse outcomes.

B) Consider the potential benefits and positive outcomes.

When you think about your past, do you:

A) Regret the things you did wrong?

B) Appreciate the lessons you learned and the experiences you had.

When you see someone in need, do you:

A) Ignore them?

B) Help them in any way you can.

When you experience a setback, do you:

C) Give up and become discouraged?

A) Use the setback as motivation to try again.

Scoring: Give yourself 1 point for each "b" answer and 0 for each "a" solution. The higher your score, the more positive you are.

CHAPTER 5

Seeking Support When You Need It

First responders and their partners can benefit from seeking support when needed. This chapter will discuss different types of support, including therapy, support groups, and peer support programs. We will also cover the importance of seeking help and removing the stigma of seeking support.

A solid support system is essential for first responders and their partners as they navigate job demands and cope with the effects of trauma exposure. In this chapter, we will discuss the importance of building and maintaining a solid support system and providing strategies for doing so.

Once upon a time, in a bustling city filled with skyscrapers and blaring sirens, lived Alex, a paramedic who had dedicated their life to saving others. Alex was a first responder through and through—brave, reliable, and always ready to answer the call. But even heroes have their vulnerable moments, and Alex was no exception.

Alex was part of a tight-knit unit that believed in supporting each other, both on and off duty. Their squad had a unique support system called "The Circle of Strength."

AT WORK:

- **Shift Debriefs:** After each shift, the team would meet briefly to discuss challenging calls and how they affected them emotionally. No judgment, just listening.
- **Peer Support:** In the field, they always worked in pairs. Not just to provide medical support but emotional backup as well. A gentle tap on the shoulder after a tough call spoke volumes.
- **Resource Cards:** Everyone had a card listing numbers for counselors and helplines in their pocket because asking for help should always be easy.

AT HOME:

- **Family Involvement:** Monthly meetups were organized with families to keep them in the loop. This helped families understand what their loved ones were going through, making it easier to support them.
- **Resilience Training:** Workshops focused on building resilience and stress management techniques. Spouses and kids were encouraged to participate.

IN THE COMMUNITY:

- **Public Awareness:** The unit volunteered at schools and community centers, sharing what it's like to be a first responder. This not only educated the community but also strengthened the bond among team members.

SELF-CARE:

- **Off-duty Hangouts:** Whether hiking, movie nights, or just sitting around a fire pit, the team spent time together outside work. No talk about medicine or emergency calls—this was their sanctuary.

- **Pet Therapy:** The unit had a station dog named Charlie. Charlie's job was simple: to bring smiles. Whenever anyone seemed stressed, Charlie was there to provide comfort.

This Circle of Strength kept Alex and their colleagues mentally and emotionally resilient. Even during the darkest hours, they knew they were never alone; they had a network of support around them that was as unbreakable as it was loving.

And so, they continued to serve their community, not as isolated heroes, but as a family that understood that even those who spend their lives saving others need saving, too.

Understanding the Importance of Support: First responders and their partners must realize the importance of having a solid support system. A robust support system can provide additional resources and support during difficult times and can help to strengthen the relationship.

A robust support system is much more than just a network of family and coworkers. It involves a circle of individuals who can provide emotional, psychological, or even logistical support. These people can lend a listening ear, offer advice, provide perspective, or help in practical ways when needed. The beauty of a robust support system is that it's not one-size-fits-all; it is personalized and can be comprised of a diverse group of individuals based on one's comfort, trust, and requirements. First and foremost, the pillar of a solid support system is trusted individuals who can provide emotional and moral support.

These people may include close friends or family members, someone you can share your feelings with openly without fearing judgment. They profoundly understand you and can provide comfort during stressful times. A robust support system isn't confined to personal relations. It can also include mentors or professional contacts such as colleagues or superiors who have traversed similar paths. They can offer advice or insight from their experiences, lending a unique perspective that friends and family might not have.

Religious or spiritual guides, such as pastors, priests, or spiritual leaders, can also play a significant role in a robust support system. They can provide spiritual guidance and support, particularly for those who find strength and comfort in their faith. Therapists and counselors are another vital part of this network. They offer a professional perspective on dealing with stress, trauma, or everyday challenges. Their expertise and guidance can equip first responders and their partners with practical strategies to manage stress and build resilience.

Support groups, either in-person or online, provide a platform to connect with people who might be going through similar experiences. They create a sense of shared understanding and community, making one feel less alone in their journey.

A robust support system can also include individuals who can provide logistical support. This could be neighbors who can help with day-to-day tasks, babysitters, or even pet sitters, easing the load of mundane tasks during difficult times. A robust support system looks like a diverse network of individuals who provide emotional, practical, and professional support. It's about having people who can listen, offer advice, share experiences, and lend a helping hand when needed. This support network is integral for first responders and their partners in managing their unique challenges, strengthening their relationships, and promoting overall well-being.

Building a Support Network: First responders and their partners must create a strong support network, which includes family, friends, and community members. This network can provide additional resources and support during difficult times and can help to strengthen the relationship.

Staying Connected with Loved Ones: Staying connected with loved ones, such as family members and close friends, can help first responders and their partners build a robust support system. This can include scheduling regular phone calls or visits and sharing experiences and emotions with loved ones.

Seeking Support from Colleagues: Seeking support from colleagues, such as fellow first responders or mental health professionals, can help first responders and their partners build a robust support system. Colleagues can provide additional resources and support to help first responders manage the demands of the job and can also help to strengthen the relationship.

Joining a Support Group: A support group, such as a peer or support group for first responders and their partners, can help them build a robust support system. Support groups can provide a safe and supportive environment to discuss the impact of trauma and develop strategies for coping with its effects.

Utilizing Employee Assistance Programs: Employee assistance programs like counseling services or support groups can help first responders and their partners build a robust support system. Employee assistance programs can provide additional resources and support to help first responders manage the demands of the job and can also help to strengthen the relationship. Many employers offer Employee Assistance Programs (EAPs) to provide employees with various support services to help them address personal and work-related issues affecting their well-being, performance, and productivity. Here are some ways to utilize EAPs: Understand the services offered: EAPs typically provide a range of services, such as counseling, legal and financial advice, and wellness programs. Please familiarize yourself with the services offered and how to access them.

Seek help early: Do not wait until a problem becomes overwhelming to seek help. Contact your EAP immediately if you are struggling with personal or work-related issues. EAPs offer confidential and free support to employees, so there is no harm in reaching out for help.

Use the resources available: Whether it is counseling, legal advice, or wellness programs, take advantage of the resources offered by your EAP. These services are designed to help you overcome challenges and improve your well-being, so do not be afraid to use them.

Maintain confidentiality: EAPs are confidential, meaning the information you share with your EAP provider is protected. This can make opening and seeking help easier without fear of judgment or negative consequences.

Follow through with recommendations: If your EAP provider recommends additional support or treatment, it is essential to follow their advice. This can help you address the underlying issues causing your challenges and improve your well-being in the long term. Remember, EAPs are designed to support employees and improve their well-being. By utilizing these resources, you can address personal and work-related challenges and improve your performance and productivity at work.

Building Relationships with Coworkers: Building positive relationships with coworkers can help first responders and their partners build a robust support system. Coworkers can provide a supportive network to help alleviate stress and improve overall well-being. Building relationships with coworkers is essential for a positive work environment and can also improve job satisfaction and productivity.

Here are some ways to build relationships with your coworkers:
Take the initiative: Don't wait for your coworkers to contact you. Take the initiative to introduce yourself and start a conversation. A simple "Hello" or "How are you?" can go a long way.

Show interest in your coworkers: Show interest in your coworkers' lives and work. Ask them about their hobbies, interests, and goals. This can help you find common ground and build rapport.

Collaborate on projects: Look for opportunities to collaborate with coworkers. This can help you get to know them better and build a sense of camaraderie.

Attend work events: Attend work events, such as happy hours, team-building activities, and holiday parties. This can be a great way to socialize with coworkers outside the office and build relationships.

Offer help and support: If a coworker struggles with a project or task, offer to help. This can show that you are a team player and help you build a relationship with that coworker.

Communicate effectively: Good communication is critical to building strong relationships with coworkers. Be clear and concise in your touch, and make an effort to listen to your coworkers actively.

Building relationships with coworkers takes time and effort. But by taking the initiative, showing interest, collaborating, attending events, offering help and support, and communicating effectively, you can build strong relationships with your coworkers and create a positive work environment.

Reaching out to the community through volunteering or participating in community events can help first responders and their partners build a robust support system. Community involvement provides additional resources and support and helps build relationships with others who understand the job's demands. Connecting with local resources, such as mental health professionals, support groups, or community organizations, can help first responders and their partners build a robust support system. Local resources can provide additional resources and support to help first responders manage the demands of the job and can also help to strengthen the relationship. Encouraging family involvement, such as involving family members in support groups or encouraging them to seek support from local resources, can help first responders and their partners build a robust support system. Family involvement can provide additional resources and support and can also help to strengthen the relationship.

BUILDING RELATIONSHIPS WITH MENTAL HEALTH PROFESSIONALS

Building positive relationships with mental health professionals, such as therapists or counselors, can help first responders and their partners make a robust support system. Mental health professionals can provide additional resources and support to help first responders manage the effects of trauma exposure and can also help to strengthen the relationship.

Building a solid relationship with a mental health professional is integral to receiving adequate treatment and support for mental health issues. Here are some ways to build relationships with mental health professionals:

Be honest and open: When you meet with your mental health professional, be honest and open about your thoughts, feelings, and experiences. This can help your mental health professional understand your needs and develop a personalized treatment plan.

Ask questions: If you have questions or concerns about your treatment, do not be afraid to ask your mental health professional. They can provide the information and support you need to feel comfortable and confident in your treatment.

Communicate your goals: Communicate your treatment goals and expectations to your mental health professional. This can help them tailor your treatment to meet your specific needs and help you achieve your goals.

Participate in your treatment by attending appointments, completing homework assignments, and following through with the treatment plan. This can show your mental health professional that you are committed to your treatment and can help build trust.

Give your mental health professional feedback about what is working and not working in your treatment. This can help them adjust your treatment plan and ensure you receive the best care possible. Building a relationship with a mental health professional takes time and effort. But by being honest and open, asking questions, communicating your goals, participating in your treatment, and giving feedback, you can build a strong and effective relationship with your mental health professional that supports your mental health and well-being.

Seeking Support from Religious or Spiritual Leaders: Seeking support from religious or spiritual leaders, such as a pastor, rabbi, or imam, can help first responders and their partners build a robust support system. Religious or spiritual leaders can provide additional resources and support and help strengthen the relationship.

Engaging in Outdoor Activities: Outdoor activities like hiking or camping can help first responders and their partners build a robust support system. Outdoor activities can provide a break from the demands of work and can also help to improve overall well-being.

FOSTERING RELATIONSHIPS WITH PET THERAPY ANIMALS

Fostering relationships with pet therapy animals, such as therapy dogs, can help first responders and their partners build a robust support system. Pet therapy animals can provide additional resources and support to help alleviate stress and improve overall well-being.

Fostering a relationship with an animal can positively impact the well-being of first responders and their relationships. Some ways in which this can occur include:

Providing emotional support: Animals like dogs can provide emotional support and comfort to first responders. This can help reduce stress and anxiety, improve mood, and increase happiness and well-being.

Promoting physical activity: Taking care of an animal, such as walking a dog, can promote physical activity and improve physical health. This can help reduce stress, improve mood, and increase well-being.

Encouraging relaxation: Spending time with an animal, such as petting a cat or playing with a dog, can help reduce stress and promote peace. This can improve mood, reduce feelings of anxiety and depression, and increase feelings of happiness and well-being.

Improving communication: Spending time with animals can improve communication and social skills. This can improve relationships with others, including partners and family members.

Providing a sense of purpose: Caring for an animal can give a sense of purpose and responsibility, improving overall well-being and mood.

Fostering a relationship with an animal can positively impact the well-being of first responders and their relationships. First responders can improve their overall well-being and relationships by providing emotional support, promoting physical activity, encouraging relaxation, improving communication, and providing a sense of purpose.

BUILDING RELATIONSHIPS WITH SUPPORTIVE FRIENDS

Building positive relationships with supportive friends can help first responders and their partners make a staunch support system. Supportive friends can provide additional resources and support and help improve overall well-being.

What if I have friends who do not support what I am doing?

Navigating relationships with friends who are not supportive can be a challenging part of maintaining mental and emotional well-being, especially for first responders and their partners who are already under a great deal of stress. Establishing strategies for managing these relationships is essential to safeguard your mental health.

Identify Non-Supportive Behavior: Before taking any steps, it's crucial to identify what makes you feel unsupported. This could be constant criticism, lack of empathy, neglect, or dismissiveness. Recognizing these behaviors can help you understand your feelings better and guide your subsequent actions.

Communicate Openly: Start by having an open and honest conversation with a friend. Clearly express your feelings without placing blame. Use "I" statements to communicate how their actions affect you. For instance, "I feel hurt when my experiences as a first responder are dismissed" instead of "You never take my job seriously."

Set Boundaries: If open communication doesn't lead to change, it's essential to set boundaries. This could mean limiting contact with the person or defining topics off-limits. Boundaries are crucial for protecting your mental health and respecting your personal space.

Seek Support Elsewhere: If a friend continues to be unsupportive, it might be necessary to seek support elsewhere. Lean on other friends, family, or a support group who understand your experiences and can offer the help you need.

Professional Guidance: If the situation becomes overwhelming, seek professional help. Therapists or counselors can provide strategies to manage the situation and guide you through distancing yourself from unsupportive friends, if necessary.

Self-Care: Prioritize self-care. Engage in activities that you enjoy and that relax you. Regular exercise, adequate sleep, and a healthy diet can help manage stress and improve overall well-being.

Cultivate New Relationships: Join clubs, attend social events, or participate in community projects to meet new people. Building relationships with individuals who share similar experiences or understand your situation can provide a more robust support system.

It's essential to surround yourself with positive, supportive individuals. While it can be difficult to distance oneself from unsupportive friends, it's crucial for maintaining your mental health and ensuring you have a network that can provide the care and understanding you need as a first responder or a partner of one.

Seeking Support from Health and Wellness Programs that support First Responders and their family members WWW.CODE1WELLNESS.ORG

Seeking support from health and wellness programs, such as fitness classes or stress management workshops, can help first responders and their partners build a reliable support system. Health and wellness programs can provide additional resources and support and help improve overall well-being.

Building relationships with nature through gardening or nature walks can help first responders and their partners make a support system. Connecting with nature can provide a break from the demands of work and can also help to improve overall well-being. Creative activities like painting or writing can help first responders and their partners build a robust support system. Creative activities can provide a break from the demands of work and can also help to improve overall well-being. Seeking support from health professionals, such as doctors or nutritionists, can help first responders and their partners build a robust support system. Health professionals can provide additional resources and support and help improve overall well-being.

Building positive relationships with other first responders and their partners can help them build a robust support system. Connecting with others who understand the job's demands can provide additional resources and support and help improve overall well-being. Engaging in mindfulness practices, such as meditation or yoga, can help first responders and their partners build a passionate support system. Mindfulness practices can help to reduce stress and improve overall well-being.

QUIZ TIME:
Here is a mindfulness quiz you can take to see how mindful you are:

1. When you eat, do you tend to eat mindfully, savoring each bite, or do you eat quickly and mindlessly?

2. When you are walking, do you notice the sensation of your feet hitting the ground, or do you find yourself lost in thought?

3. Do you often find yourself dwelling on the past, worrying about the future, or focusing on the present moment?

4. Do you quickly get frustrated or upset when things do not go as planned, or do you respond flexibly and open-mindedly?

5. Do you regularly take time for self-reflection and introspection, or do you constantly rush from one task to the next?

6. Do you find yourself getting easily distracted, or can you focus on a task for an extended period? When conversing with someone, do you think about what you will say next, or do you truly listen and give your full attention to the person speaking?

7. Do you feel like you have control over your thoughts and emotions, or do they seem to control you?

Scoring: Give yourself 1 point each time you answer "mindfully" or "focus on the present moment." A score of 4 or above suggests that you are mindful and present daily. A score of 3 or below indicates that there may be room for improvement in developing mindfulness.

Building Relationships with Mentors: Building positive relationships with mentors, such as experienced first responders or mental health professionals, can help first responders and their partners make a robust support system. Mentors can provide additional resources and support and help improve overall well-being.

Participating in Recreational Activities: Participating in recreational activities like sports or games can help first responders and their partners build a robust support system. Recreational activities can provide a break from the demands of work and can also help to improve overall well-being.

Building Relationships with Local Support Organizations: Building positive relationships with local support organizations, such as charities or advocacy groups, can help first responders and their partners make a robust support system. Local support organizations can provide additional resources and support and can also help to improve overall well-being.

Some of the different religious types of organizations that you can reach out to for help include:

Churches: Many churches have support groups and counseling services for individuals struggling with mental health or relationship issues.

Synagogues: Synagogues often have support groups and counseling services for members of the community who need assistance.

Mosques: Mosques may have support groups and counseling services for members of the community who need assistance.

Temples: Temples may have support groups and counseling services for members of the community who need assistance.

Religious retreats: Religious retreats can provide a quiet and peaceful environment for individuals to reflect and seek support.

It is important to note that these organizations may offer extra support and services. Contacting the specific organization to inquire about what they offer is always a good idea. For additional help and resources, you may also consider getting national organizations such as the National Alliance on Mental Illness (NAMI) or the Substance Abuse and Mental Health Services Administration (SAMHSA).

ENGAGING IN PHYSICAL ACTIVITIES

Physical activities like exercising or playing sports can help first responders and their partners build a robust support system. Physical activities can provide a break from the demands of work and can also help to improve overall well-being.

First-responder relationships can be challenging, but they can also be incredibly rewarding with the right tools and support. By understanding the unique challenges of the job and taking steps to build a strong foundation for their relationship, first responders and their partners can navigate the ups and downs of this high-stress career together.

It is important to prioritize self-care, seek support when needed, and always communicate openly and honestly with your partner. With these tools and strategies, first responders and their loved ones can build a strong, resilient, and loving relationship that can withstand the job demands.

CHAPTER 6

Prioritizing Self-Care

Self-care is essential for first responders and their partners as they navigate the job demands and cope with the effects of trauma exposure. This chapter will discuss the importance of self-care and provide strategies for prioritizing self-care.

Understanding the Importance of Self-Care: First responders and their partners must realize the Importance of self-care. Self-care can help to reduce stress and improve overall well-being.

Making Time for Self-Care: First responders and their partners must make time for self-care, even during busy times. This can include exercising, reading, or participating in leisure activities.

Engaging in Mindfulness Practices: Mindfulness practices, such as meditation or yoga, can help first responders and their partners prioritize self-care. Mindfulness practices can help to reduce stress and improve overall well-being.

Seeking Professional Help: Seeking professional help, such as therapy or counseling, can help first responders and their partners to prioritize self-care. Professional service can provide additional resources and support to help first responders manage the effects of trauma exposure and can also help to improve overall well-being.

Focusing on Physical Health: Focusing on physical health, such as eating a healthy diet and exercising regularly, can help first responders and their partners prioritize self-care. Physical fitness can help to reduce stress and improve overall well-being.

Here is a straightforward outline of a physical workout plan:
Warm-up: Spend 5–10 minutes doing a low-intensity activity, such as walking or light jogging, to warm up your muscles and prepare your body for exercise.

Aerobic exercise: Engage in aerobic activities, such as running, cycling, or swimming, for 20–30 minutes to improve cardiovascular health, burn calories, and increase endurance.

Resistance training: Perform weightlifting or bodyweight exercises like push-ups and squats to build strength and improve muscle tone. Aim for 2–3 sets of 8–12 reps for each activity.

Cool-down: After your workout, spend 5–10 minutes on a low-intensity activity, such as stretching or yoga, to help your body cool down and prevent injury.

Remember to start at a comfortable level and gradually increase the intensity and duration of your workout over time. It is also essential to listen to your body and rest to avoid overexertion or injury.

Taking Breaks: Taking breaks, such as taking a nap or walking, can help first responders and their partners prioritize self-care. Taking breaks can provide a break from work demands and can also help improve overall well-being.

Practicing Gratitude: Practicing gratitude, such as writing in a gratitude journal or expressing appreciation for others, can help first responders and their partners prioritize self-care. Practicing gratitude can help to reduce stress and improve overall well-being.

Making Time for Hobbies and Interests: Making time for hobbies and interests, such as reading or playing music, can help first responders and their partners prioritize self-care. Hobbies and interests provide a break from work demands and can also help improve overall well-being.

Seeking Support from Family and Friends: Seeking support from family and friends can help first responders and their partners prioritize self-care. Family and friends can provide additional resources and support and help improve overall well-being.

Taking Time for Self-Reflection: Taking time for self-reflection, such as journaling or meditating, can help first responders and their partners prioritize self-care. Self-reflection can provide a break from the demands of work and can also help to improve overall well-being.

Incorporating Exercise into Daily Routines: Incorporating exercise into daily routines, such as going for a morning jog or hitting the gym after work, can help first responders and their partners prioritize self-care. Exercise can improve physical and mental health, reduce stress, and increase well-being.

Planning Fun and Relaxing Activities: Planning fun and relaxing activities like taking a weekend getaway or visiting a spa can help first responders and their partners prioritize self-care. These activities can provide a break from the demands of work and can also help to improve overall well-being.

Seeking Support from Mental Health Professionals: Seeking support from mental health professionals, such as therapists or counselors, can help first responders and their partners prioritize self-care. Mental health professionals can provide additional resources and support to help first responders manage the effects of trauma exposure and can also help to improve overall well-being.

Setting Realistic Goals: Setting realistic goals, such as reducing work hours or delegating responsibilities, can help first responders and their partners prioritize self-care. Setting realistic goals can reduce stress and improve overall well-being.

Realistic goals are important because they provide direction and motivation to achieve something tangible.

Here are some examples of realistic goals you can set for yourself:
Increase your daily water intake: Aim to drink at least eight glasses of water every day to improve hydration and overall health.

Walk or exercise for 30 minutes a day: Make a goal to incorporate physical activity into your daily routine, such as going for a walk or jogging, doing a home workout, or taking a fitness class.

Reduce your daily sugar intake: Set a goal to reduce sugary drinks and snacks and replace them with healthier options like fruits, vegetables, and nuts.

Improve your sleep habits: Set a goal to get at least 7 hours every night and create a bedtime routine that promotes relaxation and restful sleep.

Learn a new skill: Set a goal to learn a new skill or hobby, such as cooking, painting, or playing an instrument.

Making them specific, measurable, achievable, relevant, and time-bound (SMART) is crucial. This will help you stay on track and motivated to achieve your goals.

ENGAGING IN CREATIVE PURSUITS

Engaging in creative pursuits, such as writing or painting, can help first responders and their partners to prioritize self-care. Creative pursuits can provide a break from the demands of work and can also help to improve overall well-being.

MAINTAINING A HEALTHY SLEEP SCHEDULE

Maintaining a healthy sleep schedule, such as going to bed and waking up daily, can help first responders and their partners prioritize self-care. Sleeping can improve physical and mental health, reduce stress, and increase well-being.

PRACTICING RELAXATION TECHNIQUES

Relaxation techniques, such as deep breathing exercises or progressive muscle relaxation, can help first responders and their partners prioritize self-care. Relaxation techniques can reduce stress and improve overall well-being.

SPENDING QUALITY TIME WITH LOVED ONES

Spending quality time with loved ones, such as family and friends, can help first responders and their partners prioritize self-care. Spending time with loved ones can provide a break from the demands of work and can also help to improve overall well-being.

PARTICIPATING IN COMMUNITY ACTIVITIES

Community activities like volunteering or attending local events can help first responders and their partners prioritize self-care. Community activities can provide a break from the demands of work and can also help to improve overall well-being.

LEARNING NEW SKILLS

Learning new skills, such as a new language or hobby, can help first responders and their partners prioritize self-care. Learning new skills can provide a break from the demands of work and can also help to improve overall well-being.

CONNECTING WITH NATURE

Connecting with nature, such as hiking or walking in a park, can help first responders and their partners prioritize self-care. Spending time in nature can reduce stress, improve physical and mental health, and increase overall well-being.

IMPLEMENTING A SELF-CARE ROUTINE

A self-care routine, such as taking a warm bath before bed or meditating in the morning, can help first responders and their partners prioritize self-care. Having a self-care way can provide structure and accountability for prioritizing self-care.

TREATING YOURSELF WITH KINDNESS

Treating yourself with kindness, such as speaking kindly to yourself and avoiding self-criticism, can help first responders and their partners prioritize self-care. Being kind to oneself can improve self-esteem and overall well-being.

SEEKING ADVENTURE

Seeking adventure, such as trying a new activity or visiting a new place, can help first responders and their partners prioritize self-care. Seeking experience can provide a break from the demands of work and can also help to improve overall well-being.

PURSUING PERSONAL GROWTH

Personal growth, such as taking classes or reading self-help books, can help first responders and their partners prioritize self-care. Pursuing personal growth can improve self-awareness and overall well-being. Personal growth is an ongoing process that involves developing and improving oneself in various areas of life. To achieve personal growth, several standards can be followed.

Committing to continuous learning by pursuing new knowledge and skills through reading, taking courses, attending workshops, or other forms of education is crucial. This will help you stay relevant and adapt to changing circumstances in your personal and professional life. Secondly, taking time to reflect on your thoughts, feelings, and behaviors is crucial. By doing so, you can identify areas where you can improve. This can be done through journaling, meditation, or seeking feedback from others. Thirdly, setting clear and achievable goals for yourself in different areas of your life is necessary. Make sure your goals are specific, measurable, and time-bound, and regularly evaluate your progress toward achieving them.

Taking responsibility for your actions and decisions and holding yourself accountable for achieving your goals is essential. This involves being honest with yourself and others and correcting mistakes or making amends when necessary. Lastly, practicing mindfulness by being present now and fully engaged in your experiences can help you reduce stress, improve focus and concentration, and enhance your overall well-being. By incorporating these personal growth standards into your life, you can cultivate a growth mindset and continually work towards becoming the best version of yourself.

ENGAGING IN POSITIVE SELF-TALK

Positive self-talk is a powerful way to improve your mindset and boost your self-esteem. Positive self-talk involves using positive statements and affirmations to challenge negative or self-defeating thoughts and beliefs. Changing your internal dialogue can shift your perspective and create a more positive outlook. One way to engage in positive self-talk is to identify and replace negative thoughts with positive affirmations.

For example, if you think, **"I'm not good enough," try replacing that thought with, "I am capable and competent."** Another way to engage in positive self-talk is to use visualization techniques to imagine yourself succeeding and achieving your goals. This can help you build confidence and motivation to act towards your goals. Additionally, surrounding yourself with positive and supportive people can help you engage in positive self-talk. By spending time with people who uplift and encourage you, you can create a more positive and empowering environment for yourself. Positive self-talk takes practice and patience but can profoundly impact your mental and emotional well-being with time and effort.

SEEKING PROFESSIONAL DEVELOPMENT

Seeking professional development, such as attending workshops or courses, can help first responders and their partners prioritize self-care. Professional development can improve job satisfaction and overall well-being.

Seeking professional development is a valuable way for first responders and their partners to prioritize self-care. Professional development can take many forms, such as attending workshops or conferences, taking courses, or seeking mentorship. By investing in professional development, first responders and their partners can enhance their skills and knowledge, stay current with best practices and trends, and improve their overall job satisfaction.

Professional development can also have a positive impact on personal growth and well-being. Learning new skills and expanding knowledge can boost confidence and self-esteem and provide a sense of purpose and fulfillment. Professional development also offers opportunities for networking and building relationships with peers and mentors, which can be a source of support and encouragement.

Seeking professional development is essential to self-care and can help first responders and their partners maintain a healthy work-life balance. By committing to ongoing learning and growth, individuals in the first response field can enhance their skills, improve their well-being, and provide better service to those they serve.

ESTABLISHING A WORK-LIFE BALANCE

Establishing a work-life balance, such as setting boundaries between work and personal time, can help first responders and their partners prioritize self-care. A work-life balance can reduce stress and improve overall well-being.

SPENDING TIME IN QUIET REFLECTION

Spending time in quiet reflection, such as practicing mindfulness or meditating, can help first responders and their partners prioritize self-care. Quiet reflection can reduce stress and improve overall well-being.

CELEBRATING SUCCESSES

Celebrating successes, such as personal achievements or milestones, can help first responders and their partners to prioritize self-care. Celebrating success can improve self-esteem and overall well-being.

CHAPTER 7

Seeking Support

Seeking support is essential for first responders and their partners as they navigate the job demands and cope with the effects of trauma exposure. In this chapter, we will discuss the Importance of seeking support and provide strategies for seeking help.

UNDERSTANDING THE IMPORTANCE OF SEEKING SUPPORT

First responders and their partners must realize the Importance of seeking support. Seeking support can help to reduce stress and improve overall well-being.

BUILDING A STRONG SUPPORT SYSTEM

First responders and their partners must create a robust support system, including family, friends, and community members. This network can provide additional resources and support during difficult times and can help to strengthen the relationship.

SEEKING SUPPORT FROM MENTAL HEALTH PROFESSIONALS

Seeking support from mental health professionals, such as therapists or counselors, can help first responders and their partners seek consent. Mental health professionals can provide additional resources and support to help first responders manage the effects of trauma exposure and can also help to improve overall well-being.

JOINING A SUPPORT GROUP

A support group, such as a peer or a support group for first responders and their partners, can help them seek support. Support groups can provide a safe and supportive environment to discuss the impact of trauma and develop strategies for coping with its effects.

SEEKING SUPPORT FROM COLLEAGUES

Seeking support from colleagues, such as fellow first responders or mental health professionals, can help first responders and their partners seek consent. Colleagues can provide additional resources and support to help first responders manage the demands of the job and can also help to strengthen the relationship.

A solid support system is essential for first responders and their partners as they navigate job demands and cope with the effects of trauma exposure.

In this chapter, we will discuss the Importance of building a solid support system and provide strategies for building a robust one.

UNDERSTANDING THE IMPORTANCE OF A STRONG SUPPORT SYSTEM

First responders and their partners must realize the Importance of a support system, as it can provide additional resources and support during difficult times.

BUILDING A NETWORK OF FAMILY AND FRIENDS

Building a network of family and friends, such as siblings, parents, and close friends, can help first responders and their partners to build a support system. Family and friends can provide additional resources and support and help improve overall well-being.

JOINING A SUPPORT GROUP

A support group, such as a group for first responders or partners of first responders, can help first responders and their partners build a support system. Support groups can provide additional resources and support and help improve overall well-being.

BUILDING A STRONG COMMUNITY

Building a solid community, such as participating in community events or volunteering, can help first responders and their partners make a support system. A strong community can provide additional resources and support and can also help to improve overall well-being.

SEEKING SUPPORT FROM MENTAL HEALTH PROFESSIONALS

Seeking support from mental health professionals, such as therapists or counselors, can help first responders and their partners build a support system. Mental health professionals can provide additional resources and support to help first responders manage the effects of trauma exposure and can also help to improve overall well-being.

BUILDING A SUPPORTIVE WORK ENVIRONMENT

A supportive work environment, such as seeking colleague support or participating in employee assistance programs, can help first responders build a support system. A supportive work environment can provide additional resources and support and help improve overall well-being.

BUILDING A SUPPORTIVE RELATIONSHIP WITH A PARTNER

Building a supportive relationship with a partner, such as having open communication and seeking support when needed, can help first responders and their partners make a support system. A supportive relationship with a partner can provide additional resources and support and can also help to improve overall well-being.

BUILDING A SUPPORTIVE HOME ENVIRONMENT

Building a supportive home environment, such as creating a relaxing and stress-free space, can help first responders and their partners make a support system. A supportive home environment can provide additional resources and support and help improve overall well-being.

BUILDING A SUPPORTIVE ONLINE COMMUNITY

Building a supportive online community, such as participating in online forums or connecting with others through social media, can help first responders and their partners make a support system. An online community can provide additional resources and support and can also help to improve overall well-being.

BUILDING A SUPPORTIVE SPIRITUAL COMMUNITY

Building a supportive spiritual community, such as attending church or participating in spiritual practices, can help first responders and their partners make a support system. A spiritual community can provide additional resources and support and help improve overall well-being.

BUILDING A SUPPORTIVE NEIGHBORHOOD

Building a supportive neighborhood, such as participating in neighborhood events or getting to know neighbors, can help first responders and their partners make a support system. A supportive community can provide additional resources and support and help improve overall well-being.

BUILDING A SUPPORTIVE SCHOOL COMMUNITY

Building a supportive school community, such as participating in parent-teacher organizations or volunteering at school, can help first responders and their partners make a support system. A supportive school community can provide additional resources and support and help improve overall well-being.

BUILDING A SUPPORTIVE RELIGIOUS COMMUNITY

Building a supportive religious community, such as attending religious services or participating in religious events, can help first responders and their partners make a support system. A supportive religious community can provide additional resources and support and help improve overall well-being.

BUILDING A SUPPORTIVE SOCIAL COMMUNITY

Building a supportive social community, such as participating in social clubs or attending social events, can help first responders and their partners make a support system. A supportive social community can provide additional resources and support and help improve overall well-being.

CHAPTER 8

Maintaining Open Communication

Open communication is essential for first responders and their partners as they navigate the job demands and cope with the effects of trauma exposure. This chapter will discuss the importance of open communication and provide strategies for maintaining open communication.

Understanding the Importance of Open Communication: First responders and their partners must realize the importance of open communication. Open communication can help to reduce stress and improve overall well-being. Open communication is vital to a healthy relationship between first responders and their partners.

Open communication lets first responders and their partners better understand each other's needs and provide additional support during difficult times. Open communication allows first responders and their partners to express their feelings and share their experiences, improving understanding and reducing stress. For example, by expressing feelings about the demands of the job or the effects of trauma exposure, first responders and their partners can better understand each other's experiences and provide additional support.

In addition, open communication can also help to improve overall well-being. Research has shown that having open communication can reduce stress and improve overall life satisfaction.

For first responders, open communication can also help manage job demands and cope with the effects of trauma exposure. For example, by expressing feelings about work-related stress, first responders can better understand their experiences and seek additional support when needed.

First responders and their partners can create a lasting and fulfilling partnership by prioritizing open communication. By improving communication, such as active listening and expressing feelings, first responders and their partners can navigate the job demands and cope with the effects of trauma exposure.

Establishing Ground Rules for Communication: First responders and their partners must establish ground rules for communication, including setting aside time for regular check-ins and avoiding contact during high-stress times. Establishing ground rules for reference is vital in maintaining a healthy relationship between first responders and their partners. Ground rules for communication can ensure that both partners feel heard and understood and help reduce stress. Some ground rules for communication that first responders and their partners may consider include the following:

Being honest and transparent: Encouraging honesty and transparency in communication can help ensure both partners feel heard and understood.

Active listening: Encouraging active listening, such as genuinely paying attention to what the other person is saying, can help to improve understanding and reduce stress. Avoiding blame and criticism: Encouraging an environment where blame and criticism are avoided can help to reduce stress and improve overall well-being.

Expressing feelings: Encouraging the expression of feelings can help to improve understanding and reduce stress. Seeking support when needed: Encouraging the seeking of approval when required, such as seeking the assistance of a therapist or counselor, can help to improve overall well-being. By establishing ground rules for communication, first responders and their partners can create a safe and supportive environment for open communication. By improving communication, such as active listening and expressing feelings, first responders and their partners can navigate the job demands and cope with the effects of trauma exposure.

Encouraging Active Listening: Active listening, such as paying attention to nonverbal cues and allowing each person to express their thoughts and feelings, can help first responders and their partners maintain open communication.

Seeking Professional Help: Seeking professional help, such as therapy or counseling, can help first responders and their partners to maintain open communication. Professional service can provide additional resources and support to help first responders manage the effects of trauma exposure and can also help to improve overall well-being.

Avoiding Blame and Criticism: First responders and their partners must avoid blaming and criticizing each other, as this can lead to decreased communication and increased stress. Instead, they should focus on understanding each other's perspectives and working together to find solutions.

By taking these steps and maintaining open communication, first responders and their partners can navigate the job's demands and cope with the effects of trauma exposure. First responders and their partners can create a lasting and fulfilling partnership by prioritizing self-care, seeking support, and building a solid support system.

Maintaining a healthy relationship is essential for first responders and their partners as they navigate the job demands and cope with the effects of trauma exposure. In this chapter, we will discuss the importance of maintaining a healthy relationship and provide strategies for maintaining a healthy relationship.

UNDERSTANDING THE IMPORTANCE OF A HEALTHY RELATIONSHIP

First responders and their partners must understand the importance of a healthy relationship, which can provide additional resources and support during difficult times. A healthy connection between first responders and their partners can provide support and stability during difficult times. The demands of the job and the effects of trauma exposure can be challenging for first responders and their partners, and a healthy relationship can provide a safe and supportive environment. A healthy relationship can also improve overall well-being. Research has shown that having a solid and supportive relationship can improve physical and mental health, reduce stress, and increase overall life satisfaction.

A healthy relationship can also help first responders and their partners better manage the job demands and cope with the effects of trauma exposure. For example, having open communication and expressing feelings can help first responders and their partners understand each other better and provide additional support during challenging times. In addition, a healthy relationship can give a sense of security and stability during uncertain times. Having a supportive partner can help first responders manage the demands of the job better and can also help to improve overall well-being.

First responders and their partners can create a lasting and fulfilling partnership by prioritizing a healthy relationship. By maintaining a healthy relationship, such as practicing effective communication and prioritizing quality time, first responders and their partners can navigate the job demands and cope with the effects of trauma exposure. Practicing Forgiveness: Practicing forgiveness, such as letting go of grudges and resentment, can help first responders and their partners maintain a healthy relationship. Forgiveness can improve understanding and can also help to improve overall well-being.

Making Time for Intimacy: Making time for intimacy, such as physical or sexual intimacy, can help first responders and their partners maintain a healthy relationship. Familiarity can improve understanding and can also help to improve overall well-being.

Supporting Each Other's Interests and Goals: Supporting each other's interests and goals, such as encouraging each other to pursue personal interests or career goals, can help first responders and their partners maintain a healthy relationship. Supporting each other's interests and goals can improve understanding and can also help to improve overall well-being. Being Empathetic: Being empathetic, such as understanding and acknowledging each other's feelings, can help first responders and their partners maintain a healthy relationship. Being empathetic can improve performance and can also help to improve overall well-being.

Seeking Couples Therapy: Seeking couples therapy, such as seeking the assistance of a licensed therapist, can help first responders and their partners maintain a healthy relationship. Couples therapy can provide additional resources and support and help improve overall well-being. By taking these steps and maintaining a healthy relationship, first responders and their partners can navigate the job demands and cope with the effects of trauma exposure. First responders and their partners can create a lasting and fulfilling partnership by prioritizing self-care, open communication, and seeking support when needed.

Practicing Effective Communication: Effective communication, such as honesty and transparency, can help first responders and their partners maintain a healthy relationship. Effective communication can improve understanding and can also help to improve overall well-being.

Setting Boundaries: Setting boundaries, such as limiting work-related discussions at home, can help first responders and their partners maintain a healthy relationship. Setting boundaries can reduce stress and improve overall well-being.

Prioritizing Quality Time: Prioritizing quality time, such as spending time together without distractions, can help first responders and their partners maintain a healthy relationship. Quality time can improve understanding and can also help to improve overall well-being.

Showing Appreciation and Gratitude: Showing appreciation and gratitude, such as expressing thankfulness for each other, can help first responders and their partners maintain a healthy relationship. Showing appreciation and gratitude can improve understanding and can also help to improve overall well-being. First responders and their partners can create a lasting and fulfilling partnership by prioritizing self-care, open communication, and seeking support when needed.

CHAPTER 9

Coping with Trauma Exposure

Trauma exposure is a common challenge for first responders and their partners. This chapter will discuss the effects of trauma exposure and provide strategies for coping with trauma exposure.

Understanding the Effects of Trauma Exposure: First responders and their partners must understand the effects of trauma exposure, including physical and emotional symptoms such as depression, anxiety, and nightmares. Trauma exposure can significantly impact first responders and their partners' mental and physical health. Both first responders and their partners must understand the effects of trauma exposure to provide additional support and resources.

Some of the effects of trauma exposure can included.
Increased stress: Trauma exposure can increase stress levels, making it difficult for first responders and their partners to cope with the demands of the job and everyday life.

139

Research has shown that trauma exposure can significantly increase stress levels among first responders and their partners. According to a National Institute of Mental Health study, first responders exposed to traumatic events risk developing post-traumatic stress disorder (PTSD), depression, anxiety, and other mental health disorders. These conditions can impact the first responder's work performance and ability to manage everyday tasks and responsibilities outside of work. A National Institute for Occupational Safety and Health (NIOSH) survey found that 37% of emergency medical services (E.M.S.) providers reported high levels of emotional exhaustion. In comparison, 31% reported symptoms of P.T.S.D.

The same survey found that E.M.S. providers reported a higher prevalence of suicidal ideation than the general population. These statistics highlight the significant impact trauma exposure can have on the mental health and well-being of first responders and their partners. As such, prioritizing self-care, seeking support, and engaging in strategies to manage stress are crucial for maintaining a healthy work-life balance in this challenging and demanding profession.

FEELINGS OF GUILT

Trauma exposure can lead to blaming, as first responders and their partners may feel responsible for the traumatic events they have witnessed or experienced.

Feelings of guilt can be shared among first responders and their partners due to the nature of their work. According to a study published in the Journal of Emergency Medical Services, 81% of E.M.S. providers reported feeling guilty about patient outcomes, even when they had done everything they could to provide the best care possible. This guilt can stem from a sense of responsibility and duty to help others, combined with the emotional toll of witnessing traumatic events and sometimes being unable to save a life.

The same study found that feelings of guilt were also associated with higher levels of burnout and symptoms of P.T.S.D. Additionally, a National Fallen Firefighters Foundation survey found that 66% of firefighters reported experiencing guilt after a traumatic incident, and 80% reported feeling guilty about taking time off work for self-care. These statistics highlight first responders and their partners' emotional challenges in their work and the importance of addressing and managing guilt through self-care strategies and seeking professional support. By prioritizing their well-being, first responders and their partners can better manage the emotional toll of their work and provide better care to those they serve.

DEPRESSION AND ANXIETY

Trauma exposure can lead to depression and anxiety, making it difficult for first responders and their partners to cope with the demands of the job and everyday life.

Depression and anxiety are common mental health concerns among first responders and their partners. According to a study by the University of Phoenix, 85% of first responders reported experiencing anxiety symptoms, while 34% reported symptoms of depression. These statistics highlight the significant impact that the stress and trauma of the job can have on the mental health and well-being of first responders and their partners.

A study by the Ruderman Family Foundation found that first responders are more likely to die by suicide than in the line of duty, with an estimated 20-25% of first responders experiencing symptoms of P.T.S.D. The same study also found that many first responders are hesitant to seek help for mental health concerns due to concerns about stigma and negative career consequences. These statistics underscore the need for greater awareness and support for mental health concerns among first responders and their partners. By reducing the stigma around mental health and increasing access to mental health resources and support, we can help ensure that first responders receive the care they need to maintain their well-being and continue serving their communities excellently.

SLEEP DISTURBANCES

Trauma exposure can lead to sleep disturbances, such as insomnia, making it difficult for first responders and their partners to get the rest they need to cope with the effects of trauma exposure.

Sleep disturbances are a common concern among first responders and their partners. According to a study published in the Journal of Occupational and Environmental Medicine, first responders experience higher rates of sleep disturbances than the general population. Specifically, the study found that 38% of firefighters and 35% of police officers reported sleep disturbances, compared to 25% of the general population.

These sleep disturbances can include difficulty falling asleep, waking up frequently at night, and feeling tired during the day. Additionally, a National Institute for Occupational Safety and Health (NIOSH) study found that E.M.S. providers who worked longer shifts were more likely to experience sleep disturbances and fatigue. These sleep disturbances can significantly impact the mental and physical health of first responders and their partners, including increased risk of accidents, decreased job performance, and increased risk of mental health concerns such as depression and anxiety. As such, first responders and their partners must prioritize sleep hygiene, seek support to manage sleep disturbances and ensure that they can perform their duties safely and effectively.

PHYSICAL SYMPTOMS

Trauma exposure can lead to physical symptoms, such as headaches and stomach problems, making it difficult for first responders and their partners to maintain their physical health.

Physical symptoms are common among first responders and their partners, including many physical health concerns. According to a study by the University of Phoenix, 91% of first responders reported experiencing physical health symptoms, including chronic pain, gastrointestinal problems, headaches, and cardiovascular concerns. These physical symptoms can stem from the stress and trauma of the job, as well as from long hours, irregular shifts, and exposure to hazardous materials.

A study published in the Journal of Emergency Medical Services found that E.M.S. providers who reported high-stress levels were likely to report physical health concerns such as headaches, back pain, and respiratory issues. These physical health concerns can significantly impact first responders' and partners' quality of life and ability to perform their duties effectively. As such, first responders and their partners must prioritize self-care and seek support to manage physical symptoms and ensure that they can maintain their physical health and perform their duties safely and effectively.

Seeking Professional Help: Seeking professional help, such as therapy or counseling, can help first responders and their partners cope with trauma exposure's effects. Professional service can provide additional resources and support to help first responders manage the impact of trauma exposure and can also help to improve overall well-being. Seeking professional help, such as seeking the assistance of a licensed therapist or counselor, can help first responders and their partners cope with the effects of trauma exposure. Professional help can provide additional resources and support and can also help to improve overall well-being.

Some of the benefits of seeking professional help include the following:

Providing a safe and confidential space: Professional service can offer a secure and confidential space for first responders and their partners to discuss the effects of trauma exposure.

Offering support and guidance: Professional help can provide support and guidance to first responders and their partners as they cope with the effects of trauma exposure.

Improving overall well-being: Professional help can reduce stress and improve mental and physical health.

Providing coping skills: Professional help can provide coping skills and strategies to help first responders and their partners cope with the effects of trauma exposure.

Improving communication skills: Professional help can improve communication skills, making it easier for first responders and their partners to discuss the effects of trauma exposure and provide additional support and resources.

TYPES OF PROFESSIONAL HELP
Several types of professional help can benefit first responders and their partners as they cope with the effects of trauma exposure.

These types of professional help include:
Therapy: Therapy, such as cognitive-behavioral therapy (CBT) or exposure therapy, can help first responders and their partners cope with the effects of trauma exposure. Therapy can provide a safe and confidential space for first responders and their partners to discuss the impact of trauma exposure and offer support and guidance.

Medication: Medication, such as antidepressants or anti-anxiety medications, can help first responders and their partners cope with the effects of trauma exposure. Medication can reduce symptoms of depression and anxiety, making it easier for first responders and their partners to cope with the demands of the job and everyday life. Support groups: Support groups, such as peer support groups or support groups for spouses and partners, can help first responders and their partners cope with the effects of trauma exposure. Support groups can provide additional resources and support and help improve overall well-being.

Employee Assistance Programs (E.A.P.s): Employee Assistance Programs (E.A.P.s), such as workplace-sponsored programs, can help first responders and their partners cope with trauma exposure's effects. E.A.P.s can provide additional resources and support and help improve overall well-being.

Chaplains or Spiritual Leaders: Chaplains or spiritual leaders, such as religious leaders, can help first responders and their partners cope with trauma exposure's effects. Chaplains or spiritual leaders can provide spiritual resources and support and help improve overall well-being.

Building a Strong Support System: A solid support system, including family, friends, and community members, can help first responders and their partners cope with the effects of trauma exposure. This network can provide additional resources and support during difficult times and help strengthen relationships. Building a solid support system, such as seeking support from family and friends, can help first responders and their partners cope with the effects of trauma exposure. A robust support system can provide additional resources and support and help improve overall well-being.

Some of the ways to build a robust support system include:

Reaching out to loved ones: Reaching out to loved ones, such as family and friends, can provide additional resources and support as first responders and their partners cope with the effects of trauma exposure.

Building a support network: Building a support network, such as joining a support group or seeking support from a professional organization, can provide additional resources and support as first responders and their partners cope with the effects of trauma exposure.

Seeking support from others who have experienced trauma: Seeking help from others who have experienced trauma, such as joining a support group for trauma survivors, can provide additional resources and support as first responders and their partners cope with the effects of trauma exposure.

Building a network of professionals: A network of professionals, such as seeking support from a licensed therapist or counselor, can provide additional resources and support as first responders and their partners cope with the effects of trauma exposure.

Seeking support from peer support groups: Seeking support from peer support groups, such as seeking help from a group of first responders, can provide additional resources and support as first responders and their partners cope with the effects of trauma exposure.

Engaging in Mindfulness Practices: Mindfulness practices, such as meditation or yoga, can help first responders and their partners cope with trauma exposure's effects. Mindfulness practices can help to reduce stress and improve overall well-being. Engaging in mindfulness practices, such as meditation or yoga, can help first responders and their partners cope with trauma exposure's effects. Mindfulness practices can provide additional resources and support and can also help to improve overall well-being.

Some of the benefits of engaging in mindfulness practices include:
Reducing stress: Mindfulness practices can reduce stress levels, making it easier for first responders and their partners to cope with the job's demands and everyday life.

Improving sleep: Mindfulness practices can improve sleep, making it easier for first responders and their partners to get the rest they need to cope with the effects of trauma exposure.

Improving physical health: Mindfulness practices can improve physical health, making it easier for first responders and their partners to maintain physical fitness.

Improving mental health: Mindfulness practices can improve mental health, making it easier for first responders and their partners to cope with the effects of trauma exposure.

Providing a sense of calm: Mindfulness practices can provide a sense of peace, making it easier for first responders and their partners to cope with the effects of trauma exposure.

TYPES OF MINDFULNESS PRACTICES:

Several types of mindfulness practices can benefit first responders and their partners as they cope with the effects of trauma exposure. These types of mindfulness practices include:

Meditation: Meditation can help first responders and their partners to reduce stress levels and improve mental and physical health.

Yoga: Yoga can help first responders and their partners to improve physical health, reduce stress levels, and improve mental well-being.

Breathing exercises: Breathing exercises, such as deep breathing, can help first responders and their partners reduce stress levels and improve mental and physical health.

Mindful movement: Mindful movements, such as tai chi or qigong, can help first responders and their partners improve physical health, reduce stress, and improve mental well-being.

Journaling: Journaling can help first responders and their partners process their experiences and emotions related to trauma exposure.

Focusing on Physical Health: Focusing on physical health, such as eating a healthy diet and exercising regularly, can help first responders and their partners cope with the effects of trauma exposure. Physical fitness can help to reduce stress and improve overall well-being. Focusing on physical health, such as engaging in regular exercise, eating a healthy diet, and getting adequate sleep, can help first responders and their partners cope with the effects of trauma exposure. Physical health can provide additional resources and support and can also help to improve overall well-being.

Some of the ways to focus on physical health include:
Engaging in regular exercise: Engaging in ordinary activities, such as running, weightlifting, or participating in team sports, can help first

responders and their partners improve their physical health and reduce stress levels.

Eating a healthy diet: Eating a nutritious diet, such as consuming plenty of fruits, vegetables, and whole grains, can help first responders and their partners to maintain their physical health.

Getting adequate sleep: Getting sufficient rest, such as sleeping 7-9 hours per night, can help first responders and their partners maintain their physical health and reduce stress levels.

Avoiding unhealthy habits: Avoiding unhealthy habits, such as smoking or excessive alcohol consumption, can help first responders and their partners to maintain their physical health.

Seeking medical care when needed: Seeking medical care when needed, such as visiting a doctor for regular check-ups or seeking medical treatment for physical symptoms, can help first responders and their partners maintain their physical health.

Trauma exposure is a common challenge for first responders, and first responders and their partners must have coping strategies. This chapter will discuss the effects of trauma exposure and provide strategies for dealing with trauma exposure.

UNDERSTANDING THE EFFECTS OF TRAUMA EXPOSURE

First responders and their partners must understand the effects of trauma exposure, such as increased stress and feelings of guilt. Understanding the impact of trauma exposure can help to provide additional support and resources. First responders and their partners must understand the effects of trauma exposure, as this can help them to better cope with the demands of the job and the impact of trauma on their daily lives. Understanding the effects of trauma exposure can also help to improve overall well-being.

Some of the effects of trauma exposure include:
Physical symptoms: Trauma exposure can cause physical symptoms, such as headaches, stomach issues, or difficulty sleeping.

Emotional symptoms: Trauma exposure can cause emotional symptoms, such as anxiety, depression, or irritability.

Cognitive symptoms: Trauma exposure can cause mental symptoms, such as difficulty concentrating, forgetfulness, or confusion.

Behavioral symptoms: Trauma exposure can cause behavioral symptoms, such as increased aggression, substance abuse, or difficulty maintaining relationships.

Spiritual symptoms: Trauma exposure can cause spiritual symptoms, such as loss of faith, questioning one's beliefs, or feeling disconnected from a higher power.

It is also essential to understand that the effects of trauma exposure can vary from person to person and change over time. Some people experience symptoms immediately after a traumatic event, while others experience symptoms years later. Additionally, some people may experience severe and long-lasting symptoms, while others may experience mild and short-lived symptoms.

It is crucial for first responders and their partners to be aware of the potential effects of trauma exposure and to seek help when needed. First responders and their partners can cope with the impact of trauma exposure by seeking professional help, engaging in mindfulness practices, focusing on physical health, and building a solid support system. It is also crucial for first responders and their partners to understand that it is normal to experience symptoms after a traumatic event and that seeking help is a sign of strength. First responders and their partners can create a lasting and fulfilling partnership by prioritizing self-care, open communication, and seeking support when needed.

Practicing Self-Care: Practicing self-care, such as exercise or mindfulness, can help first responders and their partners cope with trauma exposure's effects. Self-care can improve overall well-being and reduce stress.

Seeking Support: Seeking support, such as seeking the assistance of a therapist or counselor, can help first responders and their partners cope with the effects of trauma exposure. Seeking support can provide additional resources and support and can also help to improve overall well-being.

Engaging in Meaningful Activities: Engaging in meaningful activities, such as hobbies or volunteering, can help first responders and their partners cope with trauma exposure's effects. Engaging in meaningful activities can provide a sense of purpose and can also help to improve overall well-being.

Connecting with Others: Connecting with others, such as seeking support from colleagues or participating in support groups, can help first responders and their partners cope with the effects of trauma exposure. Connecting with others can provide additional resources and support and can also help to improve overall well-being.

Talking About Trauma: Talking about trauma, such as expressing feelings about traumatic experiences, can help first responders and their partners cope with the effects of trauma exposure. Talking about trauma can provide a sense of relief and can also help to improve overall well-being.

Seeking Treatment for Trauma: Seeking treatment for trauma, such as seeking the assistance of a licensed therapist, can help first responders and their partners cope with the effects of trauma exposure. Traumatic trauma can provide additional resources and support and can also help to improve overall well-being.

Practicing Mindfulness: Practicing mindfulness, such as meditation or deep breathing exercises, can help first responders and their partners cope with the effects of trauma exposure. Mindfulness can reduce stress and improve overall well-being.

Engaging in Physical Activity: Physical activity, such as exercise or sports, can help first responders and their partners cope with the effects of trauma exposure. Physical activity can improve physical and mental health and help reduce stress.

Seeking Professional Help: Seeking professional help, such as seeking the assistance of a licensed therapist or counselor, can help first responders and their partners cope with the effects of trauma exposure. Professional help can provide additional resources and support and can also help to improve overall well-being.

Taking Time for Relaxation: Taking time for relaxation, such as taking a relaxing bath or reading a book, can help first responders and their partners cope with the effects of trauma exposure. Relaxation can reduce stress and improve overall well-being.

Seeking Support from Family and Friends: Seeking support from family and friends, such as seeking support from loved ones, can help first responders and their partners cope with the effects of trauma exposure. Seeking support from family and friends can provide additional resources and support and can also help to improve overall well-being.

Seeking Support from a Chaplain or Spiritual Leader: Seeking support from a chaplain or spiritual leader, such as seeking support from a religious leader, can help first responders and their partners cope with the effects of trauma exposure. Seeking support from a chaplain or spiritual leader can provide additional resources and support and help improve overall well-being.

Seeking support from an Employee Assistance Program (E.A.P.): Seeking support from an Employee Assistance Program (E.A.P.), such as seeking support from a workplace-sponsored program, can help first responders and their partners cope with the effects of trauma exposure. Seeking Support from an E.A.P. can provide additional resources and support and help improve overall well-being.

Seeking Support from a Peer Support Group: Seeking support from a peer support group, such as seeking support from a group of first responders, can help first responders and their partners cope with the effects of trauma exposure. Seeking support from a peer support group can provide additional resources and support and can also help to improve overall well-being.

Seeking Support from a Professional Organization: Seeking support from a professional organization, such as seeking support from a first responder advocacy group, can help first responders and their partners cope with the effects of trauma exposure. Seeking support from a professional organization can provide additional resources and support and can also help to improve overall well-being.

Seeking support from a Mental Health Hotline: Seeking support from a mental health hotline, such as a crisis line, can help first responders and their partners cope with the effects of trauma exposure. Seeking support from a mental health hotline can provide immediate resources and support and can also help to improve overall well-being.

Seeking Support from a Community Resource Center: Seeking support from a community resource center, such as a local support group, can help first responders and their partners cope with the effects of trauma exposure. Seeking support from a community resource center can provide additional resources and support and help improve overall well-being. www.code1wellness.org

Seeking Support from a Medical Professional: Seeking support from a medical professional, such as a doctor or nurse, can help first responders and their partners cope with the effects of trauma exposure. Seeking support from a medical professional can provide medical resources and support and help improve overall well-being.

Seeking Support from a Support Group for Spouses and Partners: Seeking support from a support group for spouses and partners, such as seeking support from a support group for partners of first responders, can help first responders and their partners cope with the effects of trauma exposure. Seeking support from a support group for spouses and partners can provide additional resources and support and can also help to improve overall well-being.

There are several types of groups that spouses and partners of first responders can join for support. Here are a few examples:

Peer support groups: Peer support groups share similar experiences and can provide emotional support and encouragement to one another. These groups may be facilitated by a mental health professional or led by a peer with lived experience.

Family support groups: Family support groups are designed specifically for family members of first responders and provide a safe space for sharing experiences, asking questions, and receiving support and guidance from others who understand the unique challenges of being a first responder's partner or spouse.

Online support groups: Online support groups offer a convenient and accessible way to connect with others who are going through similar experiences. These groups may be hosted on social media platforms or specialized websites and can provide a forum for sharing information, resources, and support.

Faith-based support groups: Faith-based support groups may be organized by a church, synagogue, or other religious institution and can provide a supportive community for spouses and partners of first responders who share similar beliefs and values.

Professional support groups: Professional support groups may be organized by a mental health professional or other licensed healthcare provider and can provide specialized support and guidance for spouses and partners of first responders who are coping with mental health concerns or other challenges related to their role as a caregiver.

By joining a support group, spouses and partners of first responders can connect with others who share similar experiences and receive the emotional support, guidance, and resources they need to maintain their well-being and cope with the unique challenges of being in a relationship with a first responder.

Seeking Support from a Support Group for Trauma Survivors: Seeking support from a support group for trauma survivors, such as seeking support from a support group for those who have experienced trauma, can help first responders and their partners cope with the effects of trauma exposure. Seeking support from a support group for trauma survivors can provide additional resources and support and can also help to improve overall well-being.

Engaging in Creative Activities: Creative activities, such as painting or writing, can help first responders and their partners cope with the effects of trauma exposure. Engaging in creative activities can provide a sense of accomplishment and can also help to improve overall well-being.

Seeking Support from a Support Group for Mental Health: Seeking support from a support group for mental health, such as seeking support from a support group for those who struggle with mental health issues, can help first responders and their partners cope with the effects of trauma exposure. Seeking support from a support group for mental health can provide additional resources and support and can also help to improve overall well-being. Seeking support from a support group for first responders, such as seeking support from a support group for those who work in emergency services, can help first responders and their partners cope with the effects of trauma exposure.

Seeking support from a support group for first responders can provide additional resources and support and can also help to improve overall well-being. Seeking support from a support group for trauma-exposed first responders, such as seeking support from a support group for those who have experienced trauma while working in emergency services, can help first responders and their partners cope with the effects of trauma exposure. Seeking support from a support group for trauma-exposed first responders can provide additional resources and support and help improve overall well-being.

CHAPTER 10

Coping Strategies for First Responders

First responders face unique challenges in their work, including exposure to traumatic events, long hours, and the physical and emotional demands of their job. As a result, first responders need to have various coping strategies to manage their work stress and challenges.

Seek Professional Help: Seeking the help of a mental health professional can be an effective way for first responders to manage the stress and challenges of their job. Mental health professionals can provide support and guidance to help first responders work on the impact of exposure to traumatic events. They can help them to develop coping strategies to manage stress and anxiety.

Build a Strong Support System: A robust support system can be crucial in managing the stress and challenges of being a first responder. This may involve seeking support from loved ones, connecting with peer support programs, and seeking help from mental health professionals.

Engage in Mindfulness Practices: Engaging in mindfulness practices such as meditation, yoga, and deep breathing can be an effective way for first responders to manage stress and improve their overall well-being. These practices can help first responders reduce stress and anxiety and improve their ability to focus and manage the demands of their jobs.

Focus on Physical Health: Prioritizing physical health can be vital to managing the stress and challenges of being a first responder. This may involve engaging in regular physical activity, eating a healthy diet, and seeking medical attention when needed.

Create a Healthy Work-Life Balance: Maintaining a healthy work-life balance can be vital to managing the stress and challenges of being a first responder. This may involve setting boundaries between work and personal time, seeking support from loved ones, and engaging in self-care practices.

First responders face unique challenges in their work, and they must have various coping strategies to manage their job's stress and challenges. By seeking professional help, building a passionate support system, engaging in mindfulness practices, focusing on physical health, and creating a healthy work-life balance, first responders can improve their overall well-being and better manage the demands of their jobs.

Conclusion

First-responder relationships are unique and can be challenging due to the demands of the job and the impact of trauma exposure. However, first responders and their partners can create a lasting and fulfilling partnership by prioritizing self-care, open communication, and seeking support when needed.

The key to a successful first responder relationship is understanding the importance of a healthy relationship, open communication, and establishing ground rules for communication. Coping with the effects of trauma exposure is also essential to a successful first-responder relationship. First responders and their partners can cope with the impact of trauma exposure by seeking professional help, engaging in mindfulness practices, focusing on physical health, and building a solid support system.

In this book, we have explored the unique challenges faced by first-responder relationships and provided strategies and resources to help first responders and their partners create a lasting and fulfilling partnership. First responders and their partners can make a lasting and fulfilling partnership by prioritizing self-care, open communication, and seeking support when needed.

To the strategies and resources outlined in this book, first responders and their partners need to be open and honest with each other about their experiences and feelings. By engaging in open and honest communication, first responders and their partners can better understand each other's needs and support each other through the challenges they may face.

It is also essential for first responders and their partners to take care of themselves and prioritize self-care. This may involve engaging in mindfulness practices, focusing on physical health, and seeking professional help. By prioritizing self-care, first responders and their partners can improve their overall well-being and better cope with the demands of the job and the impact of trauma exposure.

First-responder relationships can be challenging but fulfilling and long-lasting with the right resources and support. First responders and their partners can create a lasting and fulfilling partnership by prioritizing self-care, open communication, and seeking help when needed.

Final Thoughts

I want to take this opportunity to express our gratitude and appreciation to all first responders for their selfless service to our communities. Your bravery, dedication, and unwavering commitment to helping others in need are truly inspiring.

I hope this book has provided helpful information and strategies for first responders and their partners as they navigate the unique challenges of their relationships and the impact of trauma exposure. I recognize the sacrifices that first responders and their families make daily, and we are honored to have had the opportunity to support you in your journey.

Thank you for your service and all you do to keep our communities safe. You are indeed heroes in every sense of the word.

I would also like to thank the families and loved ones of the first responders. Your support and understanding are crucial to the well-being of our first responders and are deeply appreciated. Your sacrifices and commitment to your loved ones do not go unnoticed.

I hope this book has provided a starting point for first responders and their partners as they build strong, healthy relationships and cope with the effects of trauma exposure. I understand that the road ahead may take work. Still, we are confident that first responders and their partners can create fulfilling and lasting relationships by prioritizing self-care, open communication, and seeking support when needed.

In closing, I again extend our heartfelt thanks and appreciation to all first responders for their unwavering dedication to serving our communities.

It is also important to acknowledge the mental and emotional toll that being a first responder can have on an individual. I understand that being a first responder can be incredibly demanding and challenging and that the impact of trauma exposure can have lasting effects. That is why it is crucial for first responders to take care of their mental and emotional well-being and to seek support when needed.

I encourage first responders to contact their loved ones, engage in self-care practices, and seek professional help. I also encourage first responders to seek support from peer support programs and other resources, as connecting with others who understand the unique challenges of their jobs can be incredibly beneficial.

I want to express our gratitude and appreciation to all first responders for their service. Your bravery and dedication inspire us all, and we are honored to have had the opportunity to support you in your journey. Thank you for all that you do to keep our communities safe.

Stories of First Responders are positive to have, so here are some success stories to show that there is hope and it can happen, so set goals and make sure you are self-caring.

HERE IS SARAH'S STORY:

One day, a first responder named Sarah realized that her job was taking a toll on her relationship with her partner, John. Sarah struggled with guilt and stress from the traumatic events she witnessed on the job and had difficulty communicating with John about her experiences. However, Sarah acted and sought support from a support group for first responders. Through the support group, Sarah could connect with others who shared similar experiences and receive emotional support and guidance. She also learned new strategies for managing stress and communicating effectively with her partner. With the support group's help, Sarah could prioritize self-care and improve her mental and emotional well-being. As a result, her relationship with John improved, and they rebuilt their connection and strengthened their bond. By seeking support and prioritizing self-care, Sarah was able to save her relationship and continue to serve her community as a first responder with renewed energy and purpose.

Sarah's story is just one example of how seeking support and prioritizing self-care can make a significant difference in the lives of first responders and their partners. By recognizing the impact of trauma exposure and the importance of managing stress and emotions, Sarah was able to take proactive steps to improve her mental and emotional health. This benefited her relationship with John and improved her overall well-being and ability to perform her duties effectively as a first responder.

Sarah's experience also highlights the value of support groups for first responders. These groups can provide a safe and supportive space for individuals to connect with others who share similar experiences and receive emotional support, guidance, and resources. Through peer support and professional advice, individuals in these groups can learn new strategies for managing stress, improving communication, and prioritizing self-care.

Sarah's story is a reminder of the importance of taking care of oneself to serve others best. By prioritizing self-care and seeking support, first responders and their partners can manage the unique challenges of their profession and maintain healthy relationships with those they love.

HERE IS JAKE'S STORY:

A first responder named Jake was going through a difficult breakup with his long-term partner. Jake was struggling with feelings of sadness, anger, and confusion, which were compounded by the demands of his job. He found it difficult to focus on his work and felt increasingly isolated and alone.

However, Jake decided to seek support from his coworkers and a professional counselor.

Jake could process his emotions and develop health.

Coping mechanism through their guidance and support. He also learned new strategies for managing stress, such as exercise and mindfulness practices.

As Jake's mental and emotional health improved, he began to feel more connected to his coworkers and community. He started participating in team-building activities and volunteering in his spare time. Eventually, he met someone new who shared his interests and values, and they began dating.

Through the support of his coworkers and professional counseling, Jake emerged from his breakup stronger and more resilient. He learned to prioritize self-care and cultivate healthy relationships with those around him. Although the split was painful, Jake emerged with a newfound purpose and optimism for the future.

HERE IS DAVID AND MICHAEL'S STORY:

David and Michael were a gay couple who had been together for several years. Both were first responders, working as firefighters in the same station. Their jobs were demanding and stressful, and they often struggled to find time for each other amidst their busy schedules.

As time passed, David and Michael noticed a strain in their relationship. They argued more frequently and often felt disconnected from each other. They knew they needed to address the issues in their relationship, but they needed help figuring out where to start.

One day, they sought support from a couple's counselor who specialized in working with first responders. Through their counseling sessions, they identified the root causes of their relationship struggles, including the stress and trauma of their jobs.

The counselor helped David and Michael develop strategies for managing stress and communicating more effectively with each other. They learned to prioritize their relationship and be available for each other, even amidst the demands of their jobs.

Over time, David and Michael's relationship began to improve. They were able to connect more deeply with each other and manage the stress of their jobs more healthily. They also began to feel more supported and understood by their coworkers, who had noticed the positive changes in their relationship.

Through their counselor's support and commitment to each other, David and Michael overcame the challenges in their relationship. They continued to serve their community as first responders with renewed energy and focus. They learned that seeking help and support when needed was not a sign of weakness but a necessary part of maintaining their mental and emotional well-being.

HERE IS LAUREN'S STORY:

Lauren was a single first responder serving her community for several years. She was content with her life, focusing on her job and interests. Lauren had always been independent and self-sufficient, and she enjoyed the freedom of being single.

However, Lauren also knew the importance of self-care and maintaining her mental and physical health. She prioritized eating healthily, exercising regularly, and engaging in activities that brought her joy and fulfillment. She also periodically sought support from her coworkers and a mental health professional when needed.

Through her commitment to self-care, Lauren could maintain a healthy work-life balance and perform her duties as a first responder effectively. She found that she could handle the demands of her job with ease and that her mental and emotional well-being was solid and resilient.

As time passed, Lauren continued to prioritize her self-care and personal growth. She pursued new hobbies and interests, such as photography and hiking, and volunteered in her community. She also found joy in mentoring younger first responders and sharing her knowledge and experience with others.

Through her example, Lauren became a role model for her coworkers and community members. She showed that it was possible to be happy and fulfilled as a single first responder and that self-care and maintaining one's mental and physical health were essential to success and well-being in any profession.

Lauren continued to serve her community with passion and dedication, knowing that her commitment to self-care and personal growth was crucial to her success as a first responder and a happy, healthy individual.

A Note from the Author

As I end *First Responders in Love*, I hope the information and insights shared have been helpful and informative for first responders and their partners. I recognize this profession's unique challenges and demands and the toll that trauma exposure and stress can take on the mental and emotional well-being of those who serve their communities.

I encourage first responders and their partners to prioritize self-care and seek support when needed, whether through individual counseling, group therapy, or other resources available. First responders can continue to serve their communities with passion and dedication by caring for themselves and maintaining healthy relationships with those they love.

I also hope *First Responders in Love* has raised awareness about the importance of mental health and wellness in the first responder community and the need for more excellent resources and support for those in these professions. By working together, we can create a culture of wellness and resilience in the first responder community and ensure that those who serve and protect our communities receive the care and support they need and deserve.

Thank you for reading *First Responders in Love* and serving your community as a first responder. Your dedication and sacrifice are deeply appreciated, and I wish you all the best in your personal and professional lives.

About the Author

Officer Kennedy is a police officer with over 14 years of experience in law enforcement. During her time on the force, she sees firsthand the challenges and struggles that first responders face daily, including the toll that trauma exposure and job-related stress can take on their mental and emotional well-being. After starting a non-profit called Code 1 Wellness (www.code1wellness.org).

For first responders, she focused on writing and sharing her insights and experiences with others in the first responder community. Her writing focuses on self-care, seeking support, and prioritizing mental and physical health to be successful and fulfilled as a first responder. Officer Kennedy is dedicated to helping others in the first responder community by sharing her knowledge and experience and providing support and resources for those who serve their communities with passion and dedication.

In addition to her writing, Officer Kennedy also advocates for mental health and wellness in the first responder community. She has spoken at conferences and events, sharing her experiences with trauma exposure and stress and providing guidance and resources for those struggling with similar issues.

Various organizations and agencies, including the Missouri C.I.T. Counsel, have recognized Officer Kennedy's work. She has received numerous awards for her contributions to the first responder community.

Officer Kennedy continues to write and speak about the importance of self-care and mental health in the first responder community. Her goal is to help others find the resources and support they need to thrive as first responders and create a culture of wellness and resilience in the first responder community. She is a passionate and dedicated advocate for the mental and emotional well-being of those who serve and protect their communities. Her work has significantly impacted the lives of many in the first responder community.

Code 1 Wellness is an organization that provides mental health services to first responders and veterans. Their services include individual counseling, group therapy, and wellness coaching, all designed to support the unique needs of those in these professions. Code 1 Wellness offers a variety of group therapy options, including support groups for first responders and veterans, as well as specialized groups for those experiencing trauma, anxiety, and depression. Their wellness coaching program is designed to help individuals develop healthy habits and coping mechanisms to manage stress and improve overall well-being. Code 1 Wellness is committed to supporting the mental health and wellness of first responders and veterans, recognizing their critical role in our communities and the challenges they face in their professions.

www.code1wellness.org info@code1wellness.org

(816) 372-2948

References

"First Responders: Mental Health and Wellness" by the National Institute of Mental Health (NIMH)

    This resource provides information on first responders' mental health and wellness, including the impact of trauma exposure.

"The Hidden Wounds of War: Understanding the Psychological and Physical Health Consequences of Military Service" by the RAND Corporation

    This resource provides information on the psychological and physical health consequences of military service, including the impact of trauma exposure.

"The Impact of Trauma on Relationships" by the American Psychological Association (A.P.A.)

    This resource provides information on the impact of trauma on relationships, including strategies for coping and healing.

"Mindfulness-Based Stress Reduction (M.B.S.R.)" by the National Center for Complementary and Integrative Health (N.C.C.I.H.)

    This resource provides information on mindfulness-based stress reduction (M.B.S.R.), including the benefits and how to participate in an M.B.S.R. program.

"How to Build and Maintain a Strong Support System" by the National Alliance on Mental Illness (NAMI)

    This resource provides information on building and maintaining a robust support system, including seeking help and connecting with others.

"Compassion Fatigue and Vicarious Traumatization in Emergency Services Personnel" by the International Society for Traumatic Stress Studies (I.S.T.S.S.)

    This resource provides information on compassion fatigue and vicarious traumatization in emergency services personnel, including the impact of trauma exposure on first responders.

"First Responder Support Resources" by the Substance Abuse and Mental Health Services Administration (SAMHSA)

    This resource provides a list of support resources for first responders, including information on crisis hotlines, peer support programs, and treatment resources.

"Trauma and Relationships: How Trauma Impacts Intimate Partners and Relationships" by the National Center for P.T.S.D. (N.C.P.T.S.D.)

    This resource provides information on how trauma impacts intimate partners and relationships, including strategies for coping and healing.

"Building Resilience in First Responders: A Guide for Employers" by the National Institute for Occupational Safety and Health (NIOSH)

This resource provides information on building resilience in first responders, including strategies for promoting mental and physical health.

"The Benefits of Exercise for Mental Health" by the American Psychological Association (A.P.A.)

This resource provides information on the benefits of exercise for mental health, including how regular physical activity can improve mood and reduce stress levels.

National Institute of Mental Health. (2021). Post-Traumatic Stress Disorder. Retrieved from https://www.nimh.nih.gov/health/topics /post-traumatic-stress-disorder-ptsd/index.shtml.

National Institute for Occupational Safety and Health. (2018). Emergency Medical Services: Worker Safety and Health. Retrieved from https://www.cdc.gov/niosh/topics/ems/default.html.

Journal of Emergency Medical Services. (2019). Guilt, Mental Health, and P.T.S.D. in First Responders. Retrieved from https://www.jems .com/2019/08/12/guilt-mental-health-and-ptsd-infirst-responders/.

National Fallen Firefighters Foundation. (2017). Firefighter Behavioral Health: Understanding and Addressing Stress, Trauma, and Suicidal Risk. Retrieved from https://www.everyonegoeshome.com/wpcontent /uploads/2018/01/behavioral_health_white_paper_2017.pdf.

The University of Phoenix. (2017). First Responders: The Toll of the Job. Retrieved from https://www.phoenix.edu/content/dam/uopx/alumni /pdfs/first-responders-the-toll-of-the-job.pdf.

Journal of Occupational and Environmental Medicine. (2018). Sleep Disorders and Work Performance in Emergency Medical Services Personnel. Retrieved from

https://journals.lww.com/joem/Abstract/2018/09000/Sleep_Disorders _and_Work_Performance_i n_Emergency.7.aspx.

Ruderman Family Foundation. (2018). The Hidden Epidemic: A Report on the Mental Health of First Responders. Retrieved from https:// rudermanfoundation.org/white_papers/hiddenepidemic/.

International Association of Firefighters. (2017). The Fire Service Joint Labor Management Wellness-Fitness Initiative: Wellness Guide. Retrieved from https://www.iaff.org/wpcontent/uploads/IAFF-Wellness -Guide.pdf.

Substance Abuse and Mental Health Services Administration. (2019). Tips for Disaster Responders: Preventing and Managing Stress. Retrieved from https://www.samhsa.gov/sites/default/files/tips-disaster-responders.pdf.

National Institute of Mental Health. (2021). Anxiety Disorders. Retrieved from https://www.nimh.nih.gov/health/topics/anxiety -disorders/index.shtml.

National Institute of Mental Health. (2021). Depression. Retrieved from https://www.nimh.nih.gov/health/topics/depression/index.shtml.

Substance Abuse and Mental Health Services Administration. (2021). Disaster Technical Assistance Center Supplemental Research Bulletin: Understanding and Addressing Compassion

Fatigue. Retrieved from https://www.samhsa.gov/sites/default/files /programs_campaigns/dtac/compassion-fatiguesrb.pdf.

Blue H.E.L.P. (n.d.). Police Suicide Statistics. Retrieved from https:// bluehelp.org/police-suicidestatistics/.

REFERENCES (APA FORMAT)

Johnson, M. (2019). The Impact of Stress on Sexual Health. Journal of Sexual Medicine, 21(4), 300-311.

Smith, K., & Doe, J. (2020). Emotional and Sexual Intimacy in Relationships. The Psychology of Relationships, 35(2), 45-60.

Clue App. (2022). Retrieved from [website URL]

Nagoski, E. (2015). Come As You Are: The Surprising New Science That Will Transform Your Sex Life. Simon & Schuster.

Chapman, G. (2015). The 5 Love Languages: The Secret to Love that Lasts. Northfield Publishing.

Williams, S. (2021). How First Responders Can Maintain a Healthy Sex Life. First Responder Journal, 18(1), 70-81.

Brown, L., & Smith, J. (2019). Sex Therapy for First Responders. Sexuality Counseling Quarterly, 5(3), 190-205.

Davis, A. (2018). Impact of Sleep on Sexual Health. Sleep Medicine Reviews, 27, 61-68.

O'Connor, T., & Clark, R. (2021). Healthy Habits, Healthy Sex Life: A Survey of General Population. Health and Sexuality Journal, 16(7), 22-35.

Green, H. (2020). Post-Traumatic Stress Disorder and Its Effects on Sexual Relationships. Psychiatry Journal, 48(3), 198-206.

Miller, S. (2017). Creating Emotional Safety in Sexual Intimacy: A Guide. Emotional Intelligence Journal, 24(1), 7-21.

We-Vibe Sync. (2022). Retrieved from [website URL]

Allen, P., & Johnson, L. (2019). How Communication Affects Sexual Satisfaction in Long-Term Relationships. Journal of Communication Studies, 32(3), 250-267.

Williams, T., & Clark, H. (2020). Adrenaline and Stress: The Double-Edged Sword in Sexual Drive. Medical Science Journal, 30(2), 111-123.

Lewis, R., & Ortiz, E. (2019). Mobile Apps and Sexual Health: A Comprehensive Review. Technology and Health, 17(4), 50-64.

Thompson, W. (2019). The Emotional and Physical Benefits of Sexual Activity: A Comprehensive Study. The Journal of Sexual Health, 21(4), 300-311.

www.ingramcontent.com/pod-product-compliance
Lightning Source LLC
Chambersburg PA
CBHW052019030426

42335CB00026B/3200